Computing
for clinicians

Computing
for clinicians

TIM CHARD MD, FRCOG

*Professor of Reproductive Physiology,
St Bartholomew's Hospital Medical College, West Smithfield,
London, UK.*

Edward Arnold
A member of the Hodder Headline Group
LONDON   BOSTON   MELBOURNE   AUCKLAND

First published in Great Britain 1995 by
Edward Arnold, a division of Hodder Headline PLC,
338 Euston Road, London NW1 3BH

Distributed in the Americas by
Little Brown and Company
34 Beacon Street, Boston, MA 02108

Whilst the advice and information in this book is believed to be true and
accurate at the date of going to press, neither the author nor the publisher
can accept any legal responsibility or liability for any errors or omissions
that may be made.

British Library Cataloguing in Publication Data
A catalogue record for this book is available from the British Library

ISBN 0 340 625279

1 2 3 4 5   95   96   97   98   99

Typeset by Computape (Pickering) Ltd, Pickering, North Yorkshire
Printed and bound in Great Britain by J.W. Arrowsmith Ltd, Bristol.

Contents

Preface xi

1 Some technical aspects of computing 1
Hardware 1
Small computer systems 1
Medium-size computer systems 2
Large computer systems 3
Operating systems 4
Input devices 4
Printers 5
Smart cards 6
Communications between computers 6
Networking 7
Software 8
Third generation languages 9
Fourth generation languages 9
Database packages 10
Technical aspects of clinical database systems 10
Turnkey systems 11
Wordprocessing 12
Computer viruses 12
Health hazards of computer production 13
Health hazards of computer use 13
Computing technology: conclusions 15

2 The use of computers in medical administration 16
Introduction 16
Applications of computers in medical administration 16
Financial management of health-care 17
The hospital finance department 20
Patient registers and indexes 20
Stores and supplies 21
Pharmacy 22
Patient appointment systems 24
Staff timetables 24
Scheduling of facilities 25

Personnel selection   25
General practice management   26
Hospital information systems   26
Management decisions in health care   26
Resource management   26
The influence of computer management systems on clinical data
    collection   30
Computers and management forecasting   30
Expert systems in medical administration   32
Installing a computer system   32

3   Computers as part of medical equipment   37
Introduction   37
Computers and signal analysis   37
Automated analysis of a digital signal   38
Computers and data reduction from medical equipment   41
Computers and electrocardiography   42
Computers in the pathology laboratory   43
Analysis of signals from laboratory equipment   43
Information handling in the medical laboratory   44
Computer assistance for laboratory diagnosis   45
Computers and medical imaging   45
The technology of computer imaging: digital imaging
    processing   46
Presentation of images   48
Using computers to improve image quality   48
Computed radiography   50
Computerised axial tomography   50
Picture archiving and communication systems   51
Distribution of computerised images   51
Three-dimensional imaging   52
Image workstations   52
Automatic interpretation of images   53
Computers and microscope images   53

4   Computers for clinical data collection   54
Introduction   54
Collection of clinical data by computer   55
Types of question   55
Types of response   56
Validation of response   58
The content of a computer questionnaire   60
The initial design and organisation of a questionnaire   60
Advantages of computerised data collection   62
Disadvantages of computerised data collection   65
Examples of CBMRs   66

What subjects are suitable for CBMRs?   68
Self-administered questionnaires   69
Some aspects of computer inputs and outputs   69
   Ergonomic aspects of input and output devices   69
   Siting of terminals   69
   Screen design   70
Patient reactions to CBMRs   71
Clinicians' reaction to CBMRs   72
Speech recognition   72
Data collection using portable equipment   73
Data protection   73
Data access   74
Clinical research information systems   75
   Data models   76
   Statistical packages   76
Specialised data collection systems   77

5   Computers and medical diagnosis   78
Expert systems   78
Artificial intelligence   78
Artificial perception   79
Application of expert systems to the clinical process   79
Clinical diagnosis by computer   79
   What is a diagnosis?   79
   'Absolute' diagnosis versus operational diagnosis   81
   Analytical versus synthetic reasoning in medical diagnosis   81
Methods for computer-assisted medical decision making   82
   Algorithmic methods   82
   Statistical pattern classification   83
   Production rule systems   88
   Cognitive models   91
   Neural networks   93
The present place of artificial intelligence   94
Defining the knowledge base for CMD systems   94
   The knowledge-base as a diagnostic support system   96
   Sharing knowledge bases   97
Domain-dependent CMD systems (expert systems shells)   97
Some general rules for the design of CMD systems   97
Presenting the findings of a CMD system   98
Performance assessment of a CMD system   98
   Accuracy   99
   Usefulness   100
   Transferability   101
   Acceptability   102
Some examples of a CMD system in action   102

INTERNIST (Caduceus) 103
The de Dombal system for abdominal pain 103
DXplain 104
The multi-centre Chest Pain Study 104
Self-diagnosis and self-treatment 105
Legal aspects of CMD systems 105
Is the program a product or a service? 105
Is a program error a design defect or a production defect? 106
Who will be sued and on what grounds? 106
Regulation of medical computer software 106
Conclusions 107

6 **Computers and treatment** 108
Introduction 108
The use of computers to prompt medical action 108
Critiquing 109
The use of computers for surveillance of medical action 109
The use of computers for surveillance of screening programmes 111
Decision analysis 111
The use of computers in specific areas of medical treatment 113
Radiotherapy 113
Critical care 114
Anaesthesia 114
Prescribing 114
Handicap 115
Reconstructive surgery 118
Orthopaedics 119
Stereotactic procedures 119
Diabetic management 120
Cardiac pacemakers 120
Psychotherapy 120
The use of an on-line database in treatment 121
Nursing 121
Audit 121

7 **Computers in medical education** 123
Introduction 123
Computer-assisted learning (CAL) 124
Drill-and-practice programs 124
Tutorial programs 126
Problem-solving programs 126
Simulation programs 127
Educational games 127
The benefits of CAL 128
The acceptability of CAL systems 128
The efficacy of CAL systems 129

Factors restraining the implementation of CAL systems   129
Programs for conducting tests   130
Word processing and graphics   130
Hypertext   131
Authoring programs   131
Equipment required for CAL systems   132
Distance learning: teleconferencing   133
Computers and educational philosophy   133
The present and future place of computers in medical education   134
Computers in patient education   134
Teaching computing to medical students   135
Teaching computing to physicians   135
Training staff in computer use   135
Medical dictionaries   136
On-line medical information services   136
  MEDLARS (MEDLINE)   136
  Excerpta Medica   137
  Commercial database services   137
  Institutional database services   139
  Which database?   140
Bulletin boards   140
Reference retrieval   141

**8   Miscellaneous applications of computers in medicine
and related topics**   142
Computers in molecular biology   142
Modelling of biological and clinical situations   142
Standardisation of medical terminology   143
Standardisation of clinical data transmission   146

General reading on computers in medicine   148
References   150
Index   171

Preface

Computers now play an essential role in the practice of clinical medicine.
All clinicians should have some knowledge of the topic. This book emphasises clinical applications but with enough background to enable the reader
to understand the jargon used by computer professionals.

Few clinicians need to be reminded that computers already play a major
role in the practice of clinical medicine. Information technology (IT)
budgets in US hospitals are currently set at around 1.5–2.5 per cent of
overall turnover, while in the UK the figure is 0.7–0.8 per cent. Since the
publication of the first edition of 'Computing for Clinicians' in 1988 the
pace has accelerated. Even now, however, only 1 per cent of UK hospital
doctors use computers regularly in out-patient clinics, but at least 30 per
cent of general practitioners have a computer on the consulting room
desk. But with increasing awareness of the place of computers in clinical
practice there is a need for some background knowledge of computing on
the part of all clinicians. The purpose of this book is to provide this basic
understanding of the place of computers in clinical medicine. The
emphasis is more on clinical application than the basic technology,
though information is provided which should enable the reader to
understand some of the jargon used by computer professionals.

There is a rather diffuse borderline between topics which can properly
be described as 'computing' and those which can be described as
'operational aspects' of medicine. To take an example, the rules of collecting a clinical history should be the same for both computer and manual
systems. However, these rules are discussed at some length in this book
because implementation of a computerised data collection system
demands that the rules be made explicit in a manner which is only rarely
found in traditional manual systems. Similarly, there is a great deal of
medical data analysis which could perfectly well be done by hand, but
it is not carried out because it would be extraordinarily laborious and
time-consuming. In this situation the computer not only saves time
which was previously spent on manual analysis, but also may turn a
valuable but impractical technique into a highly practical routine procedure. Thus, there is an interplay between computing and clinical

medicine which makes it essential that any discussion of the former must stray into the latter field.

The second edition is divided into eight main chapters. The first presents a simple account of the current technology of computing, sufficient to provide an overall concept of this topic and at least a superficial understanding of the more commonly used jargon. Subsequent chapters address the important groups of applications: administration; data analysis from medical equipment; clinical data collection; clinical diagnosis; treatment; and education. In every case the aim is to provide a review of principles rather than an encyclopaedic resumé of the literature. Indeed, the latter would now be an almost herculean task, with every passing month providing one hundred or more new titles for consideration.

1

Some technical aspects of computing

> Computers are now like cars. It is essential to be able to drive, but not to understand how the vehicle works. This chapter provides a minimal background of information on computing technology, sufficient to enable the reader to conduct a sensible conversation with computing professionals.

A knowledge of the technical fundamentals of computing – bits and bytes, ROM and RAM – is not necessary for the practice of clinical computing. It is sufficient to know that a computer is a machine which processes and stores data, and that it does this by performing simple basic operations at such extraordinary speed as to give an overall effect of the highest complexity. For those who wish to pursue the fundamentals, excellent books are available in any bookshop or public library.*

Here the hardware and software of clinical computing systems will be reviewed from the point of view of a clinician or manager who is faced with choosing a system.

Hardware

For the purposes of this discussion, systems will be divided into small, medium and large.

Small computer systems

A small computer system can be defined as a free-standing microcomputer, or even a group of microcomputers, which have no communication with each other or with other systems, i.e. they are not part of a network. Under these circumstances the choice becomes that of the individual machine.

A clinical microcomputer should be an IBM-PC or compatible machine. Excellent arguments can, of course, be made for the obvious competitor – the Apple Macintosh range of equipment. Nevertheless, the PC is the nearest thing to a 'standard' so far achieved in the whole field of com-

---

* An excellent book written with healthcare professionals in mind is *Basic Anatomy and Physiology of Computers* by Ian Clark (Royal Society of Medicine Services Limited, 1992).

puting. All of these machines are virtually identical and can run the same, familiar software packages.

The specifications of the PC will depend upon the intended use.*

The choice of manufacturer must also be addressed. There are many possible answers to this question including the following: (1) IBM; (2) the cheapest machine available after inspection of the advertising pages of computer magazines; (3) the machine which is currently in use; (4) the machine which is best supported by the manufacturer/dealer; (5) the machine which has been recommended for general use within an institution. The final choice should take into consideration all these points. It is reassuring to know that, given the maturity and competitiveness of the current market, it is difficult to make a mistake. Most would agree that, subject to minor and usually easily corrected problems, all systems are the same.

Medium-size computer systems

The dividing line between small and medium-sized systems lies in the ability to communicate: if the individual computer communicates directly with other computers, then the system as a whole can be described as medium-sized. This is probably the most important group for clinical computing and is the one most likely to be found in practice.

There are two main types of multi-user computer system. The first and more traditional is that in which a powerful central machine communicates with a number of 'dumb' terminals. The minicomputers such as those produced by IBM, DEC, Data General and others are of this type. The second and increasingly popular type is the network in which the individual workstations are all microcomputers, i.e. have their own 'intelligence'. One of the machines in the network, usually the most powerful, acts as the 'file-server'. The file-server has a large central memory for both data and programs. In actual use the individual microcomputers will download a program from the file-server, together with data relevant to the current task, such as the records of an individual patient.

The choice between a centralised system or a network is usually determined by the supplier of the overall system, and his decision will often be based on the software which is to be run. Until fairly recently most sophisticated clinical software was designed to run on centralised systems (i.e. minicomputers) and this dictated the choice of hardware. However, with the increasing efficiency of networking software there is a shift of emphasis towards the network of microcomputers. Some clinical systems can now run in either environment.

---

* Advances in the performance of hardware are still so rapid that it would be foolish to give specific recommendations in a book. Readers should consult current computer magazines.

The arguments for a centralised system as opposed to a network are complex, not least because the supposed deficiencies of one or the other are usually rapidly corrected as a result of competition. At one time cost was considered to be a major factor: expensive minis versus cheap micros. Today the price difference (and technical difference) between a mini and a powerful file-server may be small, especially in the light of the fact that the dumb terminals of the mini have become extremely cheap.

An important feature is the speed and flexibility of a multi-user system. If there are many simultaneous users of a centralised system there can be a severe loss of performance and very slow responses to commands. By contrast, the speed of the workstations within a network is that of the individual machine. Exchange of data with the file-server takes up very little time.

To further confuse the choice between a centralised versus a networked system, there are now a number of hybrid systems. The eventual choice will usually reside with the supplier of a total package. If both approaches are feasible within the same package, this author would probably choose the network, if only because this offers rather greater flexibility for the later correction of initial errors: installation of a larger disk in the file-server is less dramatic than the same task in a traditional minicomputer.

Large computer systems

Large systems are always of the centralised type with multiple terminals, often 50 or more. They differ only in size and not in basic structure from medium-sized systems of the same type. Usually they are supplied by IBM, ICL or other makers of 'mainframe' computers. Most clinical systems, other than those used in administration and finance, will be of the small or medium type. A large system would be used only on a time-sharing basis with other activities.

The clinical user is very unlikely to be involved in the detailed specification of a large system. This will be a high level technical and managerial task. However, the clinical user should be warned against committing all their requirements and resources to large shared facilities such as the typical 'regional mainframe'. On occasion such machines appear to be operated by professionals who attempt to constrain the application to the machine rather than vice versa. A dedicated medium-size machine is usually a much better choice than a fraction of a larger system. This does not alter the fact that communications to larger systems (e.g. between a clinical system and a patient administration system) are usually essential.

Operating systems

Operating systems are the fixed set of instructions responsible for general management of the computer and its relationship with various peripheral devices. Many computer manufacturers have their own proprietary operating system, a major cause of incompatibility between different machines, especially with mainframe and large minicomputers. However, there is a slow move towards universal standards. With microcomputers there is much more standardisation; centring around DOS (MS-DOS), UNIX and the Apple Macintosh OS. Of these, many computer professionals tend to favour UNIX. Much emphasis is now placed on the graphical user interface (GUI) as exemplified by Microsoft Windows for DOS systems and XWindows for UNIX systems.

Input devices

The most common input device for a computer is a standard typewriter keyboard of the QWERTY type, usually associated with cursor keys and special function keys. It is likely that the QWERTY keyboard will remain the commonest device for the foreseeable future. The principal disadvantage claimed for the keyboard is that it is awkward and unfamiliar for many potential users, especially medical professionals. Such difficulties are usually transient and disappear with one or two sessions of actual use. Only minimal skills are required for the typical one-finger entries of a medical interview.

Because of the apparent disadvantages of the QWERTY keyboard a number of alternative input devices have been developed and tested in a clinical setting. These alternatives include:

1. *Lightpens* which can be touched to the screen to indicate a particular response. The disadvantage of these is that they are prone to error because of under- or over-sensitivity depending on the ambient light in the room.
2. *Touch-sensitive screens* in which a pointing finger is detected either electronically by the surface of the screen or by a grid of infra-red beams projected across the screen which are interrupted by the finger.
3. *Optically scanned barcodes* (Weilert & Tilzer 1991), which are an obvious success in other contexts such as labelling of goods in supermarkets. In a medical setting barcodes can be of great value for recording simple and highly repetitive information such as patient identification: labels can be prepared for attachment to record folders, requests for special examinations, prescriptions etc. Barcodes are less successful when used as the medium for more complex functions such as a clinical questionnaire.

4. *Optical mark readers*. Red light is used to determine the presence or absence of markers (lines, ticks, filled boxes) in predetermined positions on a sheet of paper.
5. *The 'mouse'*. This is supplied with many microcomputer systems and is a device which can be moved by hand on the surface of a desk to manipulate symbols on the computer screen, such as pointing to and selecting items from a menu.
6. *A specialised keyboard* including keys which, for example, select 'yes' or 'no' or a number from a list. Some of these can be quite elaborate, using a detailed overlay on a graphics tablet: a pen can then be used to tick the most appropriate response. Graphic tablets which can recognise handwriting are available but are unlikely to have much impact in the near future.

All the entry devices are often associated with screen menus, lists of items from which the user can make a selection by simply moving the screen cursor and typing 'return'. Graphical entry is increasingly used, with small images ('icons') to specify commands.

The attractive non-keyboard devices all suffer from one major disadvantage, which is that they **must** be associated with a normal keyboard for entry of discursive information such as names, addresses, names of obscure diseases, remarks etc. Given that a keyboard will be present anyway there seems little reason not to use it for all functions – a conclusion which is well-supported by any review of actual systems.

The perfect input device would, of course, be one that understood human speech (Bergeron & Locke 1990). Despite much effort, this is one aspect of computer technology which has advanced relatively slowly. There is some interest in special 'hands-off' situations: performing operations or examining pathology specimens. However, hearing and vision, though superficially the simplest and most universal of human attributes, have proved formidably difficult to emulate with a machine.

Printers

For many clinical systems, in which the printing needs are patient notes, reports etc., a dot-matrix printer is adequate. The size, speed and quality of print are not especially important; the major factor affecting the latter is the freshness of the print ribbon which is strictly under the control of the user. The one feature which **always** proves to be important in a clinical setting is noise, and, if there is anything to choose at all, the quietest printer should be selected.

If multiple workstations share the same printer, or if higher quality is required for wordprocessing etc., then a laser printer should be selected. Laser printers have every possible advantage (quality, speed, ease of use) provided that the cost can be met. At present this is just over double that of a dot-matrix printer of similar general specification.

Smart cards

These credit-card size devices have a promising future for identification and clinical records carried by the individual patient. There are three main types. Magnetic stripe cards are cheap but can only store small amounts of data. Optical cards store data as pits in a film, written and read by laser beam; capacity is 2 megabytes and upwards (Drexler Corporation). Integrated circuit (IC) cards have both memory and a processor. The earlier types of IC cards, developed in France, depended on metallic contacts for power and communication. More recent types (GEC) work without contacts simply by placing on a read/write unit (Walsworth-Bell & Horsley 1988). Smart cards should be of practical value in situations in which the patient proceeds through a structured sequence of events, involving different professionals on different sites. Examples include management of diabetics, antenatal care and investigative units. At the present time their use is limited by the fact that there are several different and incompatible types of card and reader; only when the technology becomes standardised will Smart cards have any impact on actual practice. Furthermore, the readers would have to be widely available (indeed universal), otherwise the patient would still need a paper duplicate.

Communications between computers

With the exception of computers which form an integral part of diagnostic equipment, all computers used in medicine must be capable of communication.* As a broad generalisation (with *many* exceptions), communications on a single site are carried over fixed wires dedicated to that specific purpose, whereas communications over longer distances are carried on telephone lines or similar public carrier services (Table 1.1). A fixed wire has the obvious advantages of better quality, higher speed and security; the disadvantage is the relatively high cost for a given length, which means that it may be practical for a building or city block, but becomes too expensive over longer distances.

Communication over longer distances is usually achieved via telephone lines. This is obviously universal and cheap, but until recently has been slow, insecure and subject to 'noise'. Using an acoustic or direct-connect modem the rate of transmission is described as the Baud rate, where 1 Baud is one bit per second, and 10 Baud is roughly equivalent to

---

* An excellent and easily understood guide to this complex topic is *The Casebook of Computer Communications* available from CASE Ltd, PO Box 254, Caxton Way, Watford, Herts WD1 8XH, UK.

Table 1.1. A comparison of rates of transmission by a number of currently available systems

Technology	Baud rate (bits per second)
Telephone line	300
Two-wire modem link	9600
Digital public network	64×10^3
Twisted-pair wire	1×10^6
Coaxial cable	60×10^6
Optical fibre	144×10^6

Twisted pairs are the standard wiring for telephones. The slower rates shown apply when they are used with an acoustic modem, the faster rates when there is direct electronic connection. The digital public network sends data as 'packets' of bytes ('packet switching'). Thus, many users can share the same telephone 'line' (wire, microwave circuit etc.), yielding a fast, cheap service. This is the basis of TELENET and TYMNET in the US and TELECOM GOLD in the UK. The introduction of ISDN (Integrated Services Digital Network) is a major advance. Coaxial cable (a single wire surrounded by a metal-shielded plastic jacket) can be used for a 'baseband' network supporting a single channel, or a 'broadband' network supporting multiple channels.

one printed character per second. The smallest (and cheapest) modems operate at 300 Baud, but rates as high as 9600 are becoming common (the V32 standard). A page of double-spaced typing (e.g. a clinical record) might include 1500 characters which, with the addition of control bits, would be transmitted in 12.5 seconds on a typical 1200 Baud link.

There is rapidly increasing use of ordinary telephone lines for electronic data transmission ('data-over-voice' or 'grapevine'). The current situation is confused by the existence of several different systems and standards, but a progressive move is expected to a universal system of communication – the Integrated Services Digital Network (ISDN). In the UK British Telecom launched ISDN2 in mid-1990, allowing data exchange at 64 kbits per second.

Communication is not simply a matter of cabling technology but also of establishing links between systems from different manufacturers with different internal protocols. Each major vendor has its own internal standards (for example SNA for IBM, DNA for DEC, IPA for ICL) but these standards are generally incompatible. Much effort is currently being devoted to the development of a set of common protocols, the Open Systems Interconnect (OSI) standards.

Networking

Most computer applications demand that several users must have access to the system, often at the same time and from different sites. This can be achieved by either multiplexing, time-sharing, or networking. Many systems share elements of all these approaches. Multiplexing is the simplest approach. Only one terminal at a time is linked to the central processor and the choice between terminals is determined by a simple switch – somewhat like a number of telephone sets sharing a single line.

With time-sharing, all functions are performed by a single central processor. The processor polls each terminal in turn: when a command is detected the program is run for a very short time ('time slice'), then all the terminals are polled again. This occurs so rapidly that to the individual user the operation appears to be continuous.

With networking, several independent computers share the same data. There is usually a central 'server' unit with a large amount of storage. This communicates with peripheral units each with its own CPU and local memory via one of the links shown in Table 2.1. The peripheral unit runs its own program and is able to exchange data with the central unit. Similar principles apply to the exchange of data between independent machines of similar size.

The problem of any network is how to avoid message 'collisions' with several users on-line at the same time. There are two main approaches to this: token-passing and collision detection. In token-passing the network has a single token which is passed from one station to the next; only the station with the token can enter the network. In collision detection there is free entry but if collision occurs both messages are cancelled and the stations repeat their messages. This is often referred to as 'carrier sense multiple access/collision detection' (CSMA/CD) and is the basis of the widely used Ethernet network. High-speed networking is a complex topic which is still in a phase of evolution, but is clearly highly important in a hospital setting where there are usually several different systems needing to share some common facilities.

When different computer systems have to communicate with each other problems can arise, some of which are insuperable. A major current exercise in the computer industry is the development of a common set of communication standards, the so-called 'open systems interconnection' (OSI) (Stokes 1990).

Software

Computer software or languages have been defined as a series of 'generations'. The developer or user of a clinical system will not be involved with either first or second generation languages (machine code and assembly language). They may have some involvement with the third generation but are much more likely to have a close involvement with the fourth generation languages.

Table 1.2. Some widely used programming languages

Name	Comments
BASIC (Beginner's All-Purpose Symbolic Instruction Code)	The simplest of all languages to learn and use, but lacks structure and may be slow. Commonest language on microcomputers
Fortran (Formula translator)	Designed for scientific use and particularly good at handling numbers
Cobol (Common Business Oriented Language)	The main business alternative to Fortran
Algol	An attempt to provide a common language for business and science
Pascal	A highly-structured language. The purist's answer to BASIC
C	Structured like Pascal; replacing assembly language for application packages
LISP (List Processing)	The basis of some fifth generation systems
Prolog	As LISP
MUMPS	A high-level language designed specifically for medical database collection

There is endless argument as to the merits and demerits of these various languages. Such arguments are mostly irrelevant to medical applications.

Third generation languages

These include all of the most familiar programming languages – FORTRAN, COBOL, Pascal, BASIC, C etc. (Table 1.2). Many clinicians have some personal experience of these, especially BASIC. Prototype clinical systems are easily developed in BASIC, but this language is not generally favoured by computer professionals and is rarely used in practical clinical systems.

Of the other languages, C now seems to be generally preferred and is familiar as the basis for some of the very well-known fourth generation languages.

Fourth generation languages

Many clinical systems are written in a fourth generation language, though this may not be obvious to the user. These include various application packages such as databases and wordprocessors.

Database packages

Of the specific application packages the most relevant to medicine is the database. The whole process of medical practice lends itself extremely well to this type of package, with facilities for patient record systems, screens for input and output of information, searches based on individual records and parts of records, and data analysis. For most potential users of clinical information systems the choice will consist of a machine, an operating system, and a database package. There are now many database packages available for microcomputers, the more sophisticated of which can run in a network. For larger systems the choice is rather more limited, and in a clinical setting is usually dictated by the supplier of a turnkey package (see below).

One of the most familiar of the microcomputer database programs is dBase IV. In its latest versions it is suitable for most clinical databases at departmental level. In addition, there are some almost equally well-known competitors which seem to offer the same features together with positive improvements – especially in terms of speed. These include Paradox, Foxpro, Clipper, Dataease, Access and many others. Because very few people have experience of more than one system, it is difficult to obtain a definitive opinion of the relative merits of the different packages. Nevertheless, it is likely that all would prove almost equivalent in practice. If a choice has to be made, existing experience is a powerful factor: if the unit or institution has examples of successful systems running in Paradox, then this would become the obvious choice.

Current database programs are very 'user-friendly' for development of systems, but the effort required to design a clinical system should not be underestimated. Advertisements might suggest that it is possible to set up a simple database in a few hours. This is true up to a point, but the more complex systems required for routine clinical use will require considerably more time. To take a specific example from the author's own experience: setting up a dBASE IV database to collect all clinical data in an assisted reproduction unit occupied three months of the time of an experience programmer. This is not to say that the effort is not worthwhile, merely that it may take more time and resources than are initially budgeted.

Technical aspects of clinical database systems

The underlying technology of database systems is formidably complex, both in the logical organisation of files and records and the actual process of electronic storage. Fortunately, in current clinical information systems the user is largely insulated from knowing where or how the information is physically stored. Instead, the user is provided with a database-management system (DBMS), a series of tools which make for rapid development and ease of use. These should include:

1. A dictionary of data items; this directory also includes all prompts, validation information and help messages, together with rules for the relationships between variables (for example, males are not allowed to have an obstetric history).
2. A patient-identification system based on one or more of name, identity number, date of birth or address.
3. A screen-formatter which enables the user to select variables from the data directory and format them as a questionnaire on a screen.
4. A report generator (in effect a wordprocessor) which is used to print individual records, lists, standard letters etc. This should also permit display formats such as tables and graphs of time-related information.
5. A statistics package which allows cross-tabulations (for example, select all female patients over 30) together with standard statistical analyses. Until recently every database had its own unique query system, but a much more standardised structural query language (SQL) is increasingly used.

Many users developing a clinical database would now choose one of the commercially available fourth generation systems which are specifically designed for clinical use and automatically provide most of these facilities. At least 50 different systems of this type are commercially available and the choice between them can be formidably difficult. On paper the specifications often sound virtually identical. Probably the best guide is personal recommendation or existing local practice, a key feature being the level of support available from the company.

Turnkey systems

The turnkey system refers to the complete package of hardware and software for a given clinical activity, provided by a single commercial supplier. This removes from the end-user the need to make any choices other than that of the supplier himself. There are excellent examples of such packages.

Most clinicians wishing to computerise some clinical function, would probably be best advised to seek out a turnkey package of this type. The criteria for selection then become relatively straightforward and well-understood, i.e. a working system can be seen in actual operation. That being said, the turnkey package does have certain disadvantages. The most obvious is cost, which at first sight will always be greater than that of the underlying hardware and software supplied. However, the difference represents the supplier's investment in developing a total system, which if produced by the individual user will almost certainly be **more** expensive.

The turnkey system may have disadvantages not obvious from the above. The commonest of these is that the system does not actually meet its original specification, or that the system is plagued with minor defects which greatly hamper its use. It has to be admitted that **most** current turnkey systems suffer from one or both of these problems. Some can be attributed to the over-optimism of the supplier, others to the fact that the technology is not yet mature. The truth of the latter statement gives confidence that matters will improve greatly in the next few years.

Another potential disadvantage of a turnkey system is that it may be inflexible. A system directed at antenatal care may not gather information in the format considered appropriate by an individual unit. But because a high degree of flexibility is well within the scope of current technology, flexibility should become one of the criteria on which a system is selected. For example, it should be perfectly possible for the individual unit (but not the individual user within a unit) to add questions, remove questions, change the order of questions, or alter the format of questions.

Wordprocessing

Wordprocessing must be the most widely used application program in medicine. The systems used are generally the same as those in other business and professional applications (Wordperfect, Word etc.). Some specific medical packages are available which include spelling checkers and the ability to format clinical notes with a few simple key-strokes (e.g. Medical Writer from Physician Micro Systems Inc, 2033 Sixth Avenue, Seattle, WA 98121, USA). There are also electronic medical dictionaries which can be used in association with other wordprocessors (Stedman's Medical Dictionary from Williams & Wilkins, 428 East Preston St, Baltimore, MD 21202; Dr Spell from Salient Software Systems, 4 Framingham Dr, Thornhill, Ontario L3T, 4H3).

Computer viruses

'Computers hit by mystery bug' is an eye-catching headline. The reality describes a rogue program which can be introduced into a machine from a variety of sources and which can erase or otherwise alter existing programs and data files. The term virus is particularly apt because such programs can invade an operating system and trigger changes which may not be apparent for weeks or months. They spread via electronic message systems or unofficial copies of disks. Alarm over these viruses reached a peak on 6 March 1992 with the supposed triggering of the doomsday 'Michelangelo' virus. The only major damage was apparently to the files of the Uruguayan army.*

---

* Reviewed in *The Lancet*, 339, p. 652, 1992.

Health hazards of computer production*

Superficially the computer industry might be thought of as exceptionally 'clean' in environmental terms. However, semiconductor production involves some of the most hazardous chemicals known to manufacturing industry, and the highest rate of occupational diseases, in particular skin conditions, chemical burns and eye conditions. Toxic factors include gases such as arsine, phosphine, boran–diborane and cyanide, and metals such as antimony, mercury and arsenic. The commonest cause of actual fatality is electrocution.

Heath hazards of computer use

A large number of health hazards have been attributed to the use of computers (Table 1.3), few of which are either real or significant. Particular concern has been expressed about the possible health hazards of a VDU, especially to full-time users such as office workers and to pregnant women. The main anxiety is that a cathode ray tube emits damaging radiation. Much publicity was given to the 'Sears-Roebuck cluster' in Dallas, Texas. Of 75 women in one department using VDUs, 12 became pregnant and seven of the pregnancies ended in miscarriage or neonatal death. However, numerous studies have shown that the radiation from a VDU, which is completely undetectable at distances greater than 40 cm, is vastly less than any international standard limits for continuous occupational exposure.† A very detailed review (Blackwell & Change 1988) has concluded that there is no hazard to a pregnant woman and that there is no reason to recommend protective devices between the screen and the user. Minor complaints (eyestrain, musculosketelal complaints) can usually be dealt with by consideration of ergonomics, screen design, and management relations (McAllister 1987). Epileptic fits due to flashing lights are not caused by VDU screens; the refresh rate (50 Hz) is greater than the rate which can stimulate a fit (10 Hz).

Another common concern is 'repetitive strain injury' (RSI), a tenosynovitis of the wrist brought on by many types of work. The threat of RSI to keyboard users has probably been greatly exaggerated (Barton 1989), and can usually be totally avoided by attention to simple ergonomic principles.

---

* *Semiconductor Industry Study.* State of California, Department of Industrial Relations, Division of Occupational Safety and Health, Task Force on Electronics Industry, Sacramento, California USA, 1981.
† Health & Safety Executive (1986) *Working with VDUs.* HMSO, London. This document also gives good advice on general ergonomic aspects of computer terminals including seating, posture, etc.

Table 1.3. Health hazards which have been attributed to computer use (modified from the April 1989 issue of *Practical Computing*). Given a certain amount of common sense, none of these is of any significance in the office or clinical environment. A review of Health & Safety requirements for VDUs appeared in the July 1993 issue of *Personal Computer World* (p. 374).

General aches and pains (e.g. headaches, visual fatigue, nausea, eyestrain, bodily fatigue, neck and backaches, arm and wrist aches). CAUSE: screen brilliance, character size and style; level of lighting, noise, temperature and humidity; working posture and working patterns.

Stress (psychological and physical). CAUSE: uncomfortable working position and unpleasant work patterns. NB: chronic stress can have a direct role in 'producing' diseases like ulcers and aggravating other complaints like asthma. It can also aggravate psychosomatic conditions and indirectly cause problems, such as making someone smoke more and thus increase the risk of cancer.

Vision problems Some computer operators wearing contact lenses, bifocals or multifocals may encounter problems.

Repetitive strain injury and tenosynovitis. CAUSE: badly-designed keyboards; uncomfortable working posture, particularly for arms, wrists and hands. Insufficient breaks in work routine.

Damage to hearing (including deafness and tinnitus – a ringing sound in the head). CAUSE: exposure to excessive noise, such as loud printers or badly adjusted earphones. Exposure to pervasive background noise.

Cataracts. CAUSE: induced by non-ionising microwave radiation emanating from electronic equipment, especially monitors.

Facial dermatitis (including occasional itches to substantial rashes and eczema). CAUSE: static electricity fields and radiation emissions in vicinity of monitor cause or aggravate pre-existing skin complaints.

Cancers (various types). CAUSE: contact with noxious chemicals in laser toner. Exposure to ultraviolet, infra-red, X-ray, RF and microwave radiation across the electromagnetic spectrum.

Miscarriages and abnormal births. CAUSE: ionising radiation coming from, plus posture and stress problems associated with working with monitors.

Male reproductive problems (including loss of libido, sterility and testicular damage). CAUSE: exposure to microwave and other non-ionising forms of electromagnetic radiation.

Electric shocks (including electrocution and injuries caused by resulting falls etc). CAUSE: poor wiring, overloaded sockets and/or build-ups of static.

Sprained and broken limbs. CAUSE: tripping over badly organised electrical and electronic (e.g. LAN) cabling.

Burns. CAUSE: electrical short circuits, over-heated equipment and fires caused by printout paper etc. being ignited, either as a result of discarded cigarettes or over-heated equipment.

Computing technology: conclusions

Though many current and future aspects of computer technology have an undoubted intellectual fascination, detailed knowledge of this topic is irrelevant to medical applications. Today the simple fact is that the power and price of state-of-the-art equipment makes it suitable for serving all the clinical functions described in this book in a cost-effective manner. There are no *major* revolutions to come in the underlying technology; most further advances will be in the application of existing technology.

2

The use of computers in medical administration

Even today the major applications of computers are administrative rather than clinical, though the balance is rapidly shifting. This chapter discusses administration but covers areas in which every clinician will be involved sooner or later – in particular the costing of healthcare through procedures such as 'diagnosis-related groups' and 'resource management'.

Introduction

Administration consists of taking resources – people, money, buildings, medicines, etc. – and translating them into patient care. (This is why the term 'resource management' has become so familiar in the UK National Health Service.) As with computing, the individual steps of administration are of trivial simplicity: it is their assembly into vast and complex structures which constitutes the challenge of management. There is another feature of computing which is essential to the management process, and that is the inherent ability of the machine to provide a total picture of all the facts of a situation at any one time. As the data are changed so, obviously, will the total picture change: as a pay cheque is cashed, so will the cash balance of the health unit decrease; as a drug is dispensed, so will the remaining stock of that material be reduced. This record of the state of a system is precisely what pen and paper (and their equivalents and derivatives) have achieved throughout most of human history. The computer reproduces this information but in a form which provides far greater speed and flexibility.

If the information provided were adequate and a complete set of rules were available, then a computer could manage a medical practice as well – indeed better – than any human. The fact that the information is usually incomplete and the rules ill-defined is the reason why computers have not pre-empted people and probably will never do so. The purpose of this chapter is to show how computers have already penetrated and will continue to take over a large part of the information base on which the administration of medical practice is founded.

Applications of computers in medical administration

There are numerous specific administrative health-care functions which are particularly well suited to computerisation (Table 2.1).

Table 2.1. Examples of administrative health-care functions
which are suitable for an independent computer system.
Some of these functions are considered in detail in the text

Finance (billing, payroll, accounts)
Patient registers (master patient index)
Stores
Catering
Pharmacy
Patient appointment systems
Nursing and other timetables
Estate management and works
Personnel (manpower information)
Equipment maintenance (Bruns 1991)

Financial management of health-care

One of the most fundamental roles of computers in health-care is in
financial management. It is also one of the few areas in which it has been
demonstrated that an increased workload can be met by a smaller staff.
Financial management will be discussed under the headings of billing,
payroll and accounts.

Billing systems

The first application of computers to medicine was the preparation of
patient invoices. This explains the apparent widespread and early use of
computers in those countries, such as the US, where much medical care is
charged directly on a fee-per-item basis. In such areas the hand-written
bill would now be regarded as archaic and, indeed, would probably not
be acceptable for reimbursement by insurers.

As with so many computer applications, the changes in billing systems
go well beyond the simple replacement of manual procedures. They
permit a level of detail which at one time would have been inconceivable
and the possibility of billing separately for minor items (e.g. analgesics,
simple dressings and disposables) has been a great stimulus to the
introduction of these systems. Thus, it is usually possible to show that the
additional revenue generated by separate billing of minor items rapidly
repays the cost of the computer installation. It might also be supposed
that the high level of detail is an important adjunct to some fundamental
management processes. However, trivial data often give a spurious
impression of accuracy: to note an aspirin at 50 cents and then a global
daily charge of $300 for hospital services hardly leads to a better under-
standing of the basis of health care costs.

The advantages of computerised billing systems for maximising income have been very clearly spelt out in the context of veterinary medicine (Kruse 1986), a subject in which the appearance of altruism need not be so overt as with human practice. Among the features leading to an increase in total fees are: removing the doctor from the fee-making process (i.e. avoiding the very human inclination to perform small services for nothing); checking overhead costs to ensure that even minor services are profitable (i.e. it costs a certain amount for the client simply to walk through the door); increasing the number of services per visit by adding specific messages to reminder letters; and automatically adding interest and service charges to unpaid accounts. Finally, there is the important question of image and attitude: 'a client may resent paying $3.00 for 10 pills ... in an envelope with scribbled instructions ... but will readily accept a charge of $8.00 for the same 10 pills in a childproof container with a computer-generated label' (Kruse 1986).

Payroll

Virtually every organisation in the developed world with ten or more employees will use some type of computerised payroll system, and even smaller organisations (e.g. the single-handed private practice) may well elect to have this function performed automatically by their bankers. There have been two main stimuli to the introduction of computerised payroll systems. First, the process is ideally suited to computerisation: it consists of a series of highly repetitive calculations, which must be performed with absolute accuracy, based on a set of predetermined rules, which may be large in number but individually are very simple. Second, the requirement, now mandatory in most countries, for deduction of taxes and other contributions at source, demands rapid and meticulous preparation of paperwork which again is ideal for machine assistance.

Simple payroll systems were one of the earlier and more attractive software packages for microcomputer systems. The disadvantages of these packages are that they do not cross frontiers (no two countries, and sometimes areas in the same country, have the same tax rules) and that they need to be frequently and regularly updated to take account of changing rates, rules, etc. For this reason, payroll in smaller organisations such as a medical private practice is better carried out as a service rather than with an independent system. In larger organisations there is a tendency towards integrated systems for personnel and payroll, since both can work on a common database.

Accounts

By contrast to billing and payroll systems, which are logically simple and therefore similar in principle wherever applied, accounting systems demonstrate an extraordinary complexity and variety. Those who believe that accounting consists of adding up income and expenditure, the difference between them being the profit or loss, are in for a rude awakening. Today it is highly unlikely that the individual private physician will ever master this topic. Courses of instruction are available but usually (and correctly) leave the consumer firmly convinced that he or she should rely on professional help for all but the most elementary tasks. What the computer can achieve in this respect, in relation to health care professionals, is to ensure that the primary inputs are well-controlled. For example, it can ensure that all ordering and issuing of medical goods takes place in a structured manner. One of the most essential features of good professional accounting is to ensure that all the basic transactions are fully recorded, and the machine can be of great assistance in this respect.

A simplified guide to computerised practice accounts

The two basic accounts documents are the daysheet and the general ledger. The daysheet is a daily log of charges made and payments received (including any relevant adjustments). The general ledger contains the same information for individual patients, updated on a regular basis (the process known as posting). On a given date the totals for the daysheets and ledgers should be equal, the whole process being described as double-entry bookkeeping. In effect, the keeping of two separate tables provides a continuous check on the correctness of the system as a whole. A computer system should emulate this classical process as closely as possible.

Accounting software packages are often divided according to function. A typical medical office will require a general ledger, payroll, and accounts receivable. The general criteria for a computerised practice accounts system (presentation, user-friendliness, etc.) are very similar to those of computerised clinical record systems (Chapter 5). More specific features include the following:

1. The system should be double-entry (balancing of day-sheets against patient ledgers).
2. Payments (cash, cheques, credit cards) should be posted on the day of receipt.*
3. The patient ledger should list individual charges, not just a total or balance forward.
4. All entries should be related to individual clinicians.

---

* Medical practices are usually run on a cash accounting basis in which income is reported as actual cash received. This is in contrast to accrual accounting in which income is reported as services rendered whether paid or not. Many ready-made bookkeeping packages will only deal with the latter system.

5. It should be possible to link to a specific encounter as well as the oldest outstanding balance.
6. There should be an audit trail for every transaction.
7. The system should provide fixed prices for every procedure, but with a facility for adjustment (adjustments might include professional courtesy, indigent patients, etc.).
8. Accounts-receivable reports must be provided, divided according to age (up to 30 days, 30–60 days, etc.).
9. The system should be able to prepare for reimbursement and insurance claims.

The hospital finance department

Management of hospital finances is a complex topic. Depending on size, such a department will have the five components listed in Table 2.2. All these functions will usually be centred around a database on a mainframe computer, supported by a network of microcomputers for reporting, budgeting and planning.

Table 2.2. The components of a hospital finance division

Payroll
Accounts payable
Cash management/treasury
General accounting
Budgeting/reimbursement

Patient registers and indexes

One of the main uses of a computer in a health-care system is to keep a central list of individual patients together with a minimum amount of information required to identify these individuals without ambiguity. Such a list goes under various names: patient register, patient master index, etc. The purpose of this list is to provide a single set of identifying data which can then be used for a wide variety of different transactions involving that patient – case notes, requests for special investigations, prescriptions, billing, etc.

At first sight the preparation and maintenance of a central list of patients seems straightforward. However, problems arise at two levels. First, it is difficult and perhaps impossible to ensure that the identifying information is always unambiguous. Second, there is a strong temptation to add information to each record over and above that which is strictly required for the purpose of identification.

The minimum information is the patient's name and hospital or practice number. The number, unless mis-keyed, should be definitive, but this is not a piece of information which patients normally carry around with them. The name, by contrast, is often ambiguous. Within a given geographic area there may be several people with the same name; this is especially common in some ethnic groups. Furthermore, a name may be wrongly entered. Many systems allow for this by presenting possible alternatives if the information entered is untraceable or incompatible with other information. The search for alternatives may be based on the sound of the name (the Soundex system: could Pattle be Patel?) or simply on switching of characters (could Smoth be Smith?). The problem of ambiguous names may also be resolved by additional pieces of information such as the patient's date of birth and address, both items which they are unlikely to forget. Names and addresses are very likely to change. This presents no problem if the change is noted and the record updated: the key link, the hospital number, still remains. But failure to update will lead to the all-too-familiar situation of the individual with multiple records under different numbers. There is probably no complete solution to this problem, and it has to be accepted that there will be a small proportion of ambiguous or replicated records in any system. Nevertheless, a computerised patient index should be much superior in this respect to the traditional manuscript lists.

There is always a tendency to add non-identifying information to the patient index, especially items which will be fixed regardless of what particular clinical transaction is taking place. Examples include race and religion, name of family practitioner, occupation, marital status, financial and insurance details, etc. A permanent record of such features is obviously convenient because then they do not have to be repeated at every encounter. However, the problem is knowing where to stop: it is all too easy to start with a simple index and finish up with a massive database which overloads the system. This is not to deny the value of such information, or the benefits of holding it on a computer. It is merely to emphasise the importance of defining the exact function of each set of data and that such functions should not be confused.

At a technical level it is often convenient to convert patient identification data into a barcode which can be read with a lightpen. This code can be attached to the patient's notes, special request forms, prescriptions, etc. and provides a fast and convenient means for calling patient information from central files without the need to key-in a sequence of characters.

A typical simple record-keeping system in a private practice is shown in Table 2.3.

Stores and supplies

Health services consume vast quantities of general and specialist supplies. The principles of computerisation of this function are no different from those which obtain in any other business. It may, however, intro-

Table 2.3. A typical set of data for a simple record-keeping system in a private practice

Patient's name, address and telephone numbers

Social Security number, date of birth and sex

Parties responsible for payment and insurance coverage

Services rendered (by date and type): number and service

Fee and insurance code number for each service

Type and amount of payment

Account balance

Date of next appointment and recall date

duce a cost-consciousness which is unusual in the health-care field, especially in the government-funded sector. Thus in a typical hospital ward, out-patient department or laboratory, supplies are ordered so that the available storage is, as nearly as possible, completely filled. By contrast, a computerised system will monitor throughput and ensure that stocks are maintained and replaced at the minimum level necessary to ensure that the store cupboard is never actually empty. The difference between the two approaches can represent a substantial quantity of materials and, in effect, money.

Pharmacy

Pharmacy services are particularly well-suited to computerisation and, after finance, are often chosen as one of the first computer exercises in a hospital unit. They represent an interesting mix of general 'business' functions together with specific and important clinical functions (Broekemeier et al. 1986; Gouveia, 1986; Tallis 1987).

Computerised stock-control has obvious and immediate benefits to any organisation which maintains an inventory of high-value goods. As already noted in the previous section on stores and supplies, a reduction of stocks to the minimum level compatible with the maintenance of service can produce a once-off saving which can often equal or exceed the cost of the computer installation. This is particularly the case with pharmaceuticals, which can easily reach values of hundreds of pounds (or dollars) per patient per day. The argument against minimisation of stocks is the savings which may be made as the result of bulk purchases (or, more important, by a single front-end payment for bulk purchases). Decisions of this type will continue to be made by pharmacy managers, but a computerised stock-control system is of immense help in reaching such a decision. The advantages may also accrue to manufacturers: the US pharmaceutical distributors McKessons greatly increased sales after giving barcode readers to pharmacists, enabling them to analyse their inventory and place orders for delivery on the following day.

There are many additional areas in which a computer system can contribute to the operation of pharmacy services:

1. *Providing a database of drug information.* The contents of most major formularies and pharmacopoeias are now available as computer databases. These provide a ready and up-to-date source of information on indications, dosages, costs and side-effects. They can also provide warnings of drug incompatibilities – an otherwise formidable task for the human physician who may be faced with literally thousands of possible combinations (Haumschild et al. 1987). In one study, 23 per cent of elderly patients admitted to hospital were found to have contraindicated or adversely interacting drug combinations (Gosney & Tallis 1984).

2. *Calculation of dosages* where this must be accurately based on body weight or patient response (e.g. paediatrics, intensive care, parenteral nutrition).

3. *Writing prescriptions* – in effect, an intelligent wordprocessing function. An institutional network also provides for direct ordering from ward and clinic.

4. *Providing a database of poison control information.*

5. *Printing of labels and instructions.* As in many areas of medicine, the replacement of simple but tedious manuscript (or typescript) is the function which immediately commends a computer system to its actual users. Such a system is so far superior to manual equivalents for labelling of medicines that the traditional approach can now probably be described as negligent. Legibility and avoidance of elementary mistakes in names and numbers are the most obvious advantages. Others include the ability to take and transcribe information directly from the database, or at least to compare this information with the instructions provided by the physician.

6. *Pricing and charging of prescriptions.*

7. *Provision of a complete record for each task,* thus permitting full personal accountability for errors, etc.

8. *Monitoring of patient compliance* by tracking the dispensing date, the renewal date, and the amount dispensed.

9. *Monitoring the prescribing practices of individual physicians or units.* A computer system can easily provide regular information on individual prescribing practices, a form of review which is virtually impossible with manual systems. The performance of different physicians in the same specialty can then be compared, both as to types of drugs used and their costs. Unless handled very diplomatically, this exercise can often lead to friction between the pharmacy managers

and individual clinicians, or among clinicians themselves. Many do not take kindly to the suggestion that there are cheaper generic equivalents to the attractive trade names to which they have become accustomed. This is not to advocate generic drugs in general, but simply to emphasise that a public discussion of prescribing policies will often follow shortly after the installation of a pharmacy computer system. An excellent example of this principle emerged from a Spanish study showing a fall in antibiotic costs following the introduction of a computer-assisted antimicrobial monitoring program (Inaraja et al. 1986). Much of this fall could be attributed to substitution of high-cost cephalosporins by lower-cost penicillins.

10. *Management information systems*. Computers can document the workload and productivity of hospital pharmacy departments; specific programs are available for this (Pharma TXrend; Wilson 1989).

11. *Surveillance of adverse drug events* (Classen et al. 1991).

12. Producing computer generated reminder charts (Raynor et al. 1993).

Patient appointment systems

Patient appointment systems lend themselves well to computerisation. One of the simplest forms is the 'appointment book' approach in which 'pages' are created in the computer exactly as they would appear in a manual system. The advantage of the computer is the ability to search rapidly for the next available slot. At a rather more sophisticated level the machine can schedule according to likely time requirements: longer for a first visit than a follow-up visit; longer for the radiological examination of a stretcher patient than an ambulatory patient. The computer comes into its own when organising a sequence of events for an individual patient; for example, in one radiology unit the use of 'time-flow analysis' on computerised data reduced the time spent in the department by an average of 45 minutes per patient (Jost et al. 1982).

Staff timetables

Clinical medicine is a highly labour-intensive activity: staff usually account for 60 per cent or more of total costs. Organisation of manpower – in effect, drawing up timetables – is therefore one of the most important management functions in health care. Nowhere is this more apparent than with nursing, which in most areas of medicine constitutes by far the largest of the various professional subgroups.

The process of drawing up a nursing staff timetable for a clinical unit is always of extraordinary complexity. A 'unit', in this sense, refers to a functional group such as a hospital ward, an operating theatre or an out-patient facility. Nursing services are provided on three shifts, 7 days a week. Staff of widely differing skills and grades are required, and the assignment process must take into account a broad variety of individual circumstances such as total hours worked, rest days, holidays, release for formal education, etc. The complexity increases still further when a series of units have to be considered, such as a complete hospital; and when the short-term needs of single units have to be met in the context of the long-term career needs of trainee staff (another feature of medical and especially hospital practice is that a remarkably high proportion of all professional staff are in some sort of training grade).

Timetables are complex structures based on the multiplication of a few simple rules and are therefore ideally suited to computerisation. Many systems have been described, some based on artificial intelligence concepts in order to optimise staff use (reviewed by Okada 1988; Brusco et al. 1993). Commercial packages are available (e.g. Sked-it available from Hewlett-Packard) but may not always solve the problem of the immense variations in practice between different units.

Despite some computerisation, staff timetables still remain a largely 'manual' function. However, there is one immense contribution which the computer can make and that is in the wordprocessing of complex tables. Sooner or later all timetables come down to the preparation of multidimensional arrays on sheets of paper. These are very tedious to construct in the first place, but even more tedious to modify and re-distribute when, as is inevitable in any large plan, small changes have to be made during the course of execution. One of the great strengths of wordprocessing is the facility for making, with minimum effort, repetitive minor changes to complicated tabulations.

Scheduling of facilities

In contrast to the scheduling of people, the scheduling of objects is much more straightforward and often lends itself well to almost complete control by computers. 'Objects' include fixed facilities such as operating rooms and major imaging equipment, or mobile facilities such as ambulances. Objects are much less variable than people: even a very large ambulance service will have only three basic types of vehicle. Furthermore, the characteristics of an object are extremely simple, being limited to time, position, and whether or not it is working. Once a system is set up it can respond much faster and more effectively than humans to sudden changes: for example, the breakdown of one vehicle can be followed by a complete re-scheduling of many others within a matter of seconds. Furthermore, a sophisticated program which controls the scheduling of operating rooms is likely to be equally applicable on a large number of sites (see Ball et al. 1986).

Personnel selection

Computers are widely used for the initial screening of applicants for health-care positions. In one instance this led to a most unfortunate result: a computer program for selection of medical students was found to have discriminated against women and against people with non-European names (Lowry & MacPherson, 1988). This unintended bias arose because the program was written to correlate closely with the performance of the actual selection panel.

General practice management

In 1994 every General Practice in the UK has at least one computer. There is an extraordinarily wide range of packages available for the general management of small group practices. To choose among them is a formidable task. Helpful reviews appear from time-to-time in journals such as MD Computing and the British Journal of Healthcare Computing. The review by Benson (1991) is strongly recommended.

Hospital information systems

Hospital Information Systems (HIS) is the term used for the holy grail of clinical computing: an all embracing system which collects, processes, stores and communicates all clinical, paraclinical and administrative information. The nearest that any present system comes to this paradigm is a collection of independent systems (finance, pathology, etc.) connected by networks of varying efficiency. Published descriptions of major HIS projects include that used by many hospitals in The Netherlands (Bakker 1990) and the DIOGENE system used in Geneva (Scherrer et al. 1990). It cannot be emphasised too strongly that an effective hospital information system must have the patient record as the primary focus (Fig. 2.1).

Management decisions in health care

Computers are excellent at supplying facts. But the question may reasonably be asked as to whether these accumulations of facts are of any real value to the end-consumer of health care services – the patient. The answer to this question would appear to be 'yes', subject to many caveats concerning the number and type of facts which should be collected, and their analysis to produce a coherent and useful picture of the operation of services.

Resource management

The manager of a health-care service is faced with a range of demands and a range of resources with which to meet those demands in whole or in part. Inevitably, consideration of resources becomes a consideration of money, and management becomes an exercise in ensuring that a given amount of money produces the best possible response to demands.

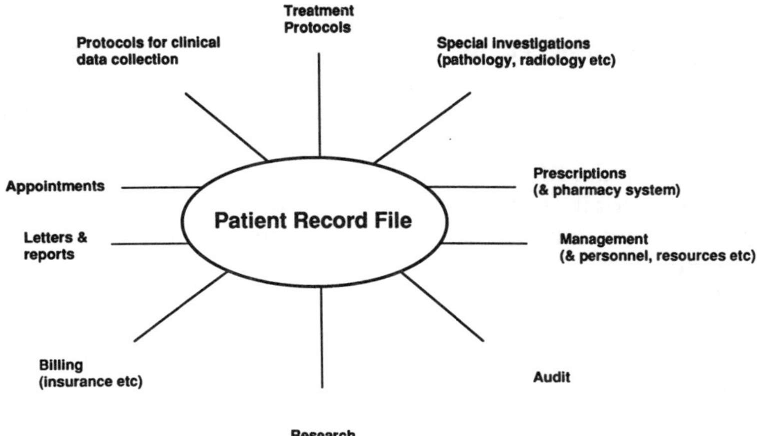

Fig. 2.1. The structure of a hospital information system (HIS). This system must have the patient record as the primary focus. All other approaches are doomed to failure if integration is the intended effect.

It is important to emphasise the major divergence in cost–demand analysis between different systems of health care: between public-sector systems and private-sector systems. The following broad generalisations may be made (with many detailed exceptions). Public-sector systems tend to be closed-ended, with the allocation of a fixed amount of money out of which resources are then provided according to the perceived priorities of demand. Private-sector systems, by contrast, are open-ended, and it is the level of demand which determines the amount of money (resources) which is available. The public-sector and private-sector systems are quite distinct in terms of management style and the contribution which computers can make to this management. They are well illustrated by the health care systems of the UK and the US respectively and will be discussed under these headings (recognising, of course, that there is a small private sector in the UK and a very major public health service in the US).

Private-sector management: the US

With some exceptions, private-sector systems are easier to manage than public-sector systems. The costs of health care are readily identified with the actual resources because they are added up and sent as a bill to the patient (or the patient's insurer). If demand increases, so does the size of the bill and thus the amount of resources required to meet this demand.

The existence of a billing system has two important implications. First, it is such an obvious application for computers that they are a much more prominent facility in the private than in the public-sector and, correspondingly, in the US than in the UK. Equally it must be emphasised that computers designed to write out bills usually do just that and nothing more: they do not contribute directly to the health care of the individual patient in the manner described later in this book. Second, the existence of a computerised billing system means that it is far easier for the manager to identify costs of procedures: for example, in the US it is possible to ascertain, simply and rapidly, the all-in cost of an appendicectomy in an individual hospital; in a UK District hospital this exercise is far more difficult.

Diagnosis-related groups (DRGs)

The fact that demand automatically generates resources does not mean that the costs of these resources cannot be scrutinised. Indeed, the wide variation in costs for a given procedure between different units, and the seemingly inexorable tendency for these costs to increase, has led to an entirely new approach to medical costing in the US – from retrospective, cost-based reimbursement to prospective pricing by diagnosis-related group (DRG) for most in-patient services. The principle of a DRG is as follows. Hospital cases are classified into clinically coherent groups that are similar in resource consumption, such as cost or length of stay. In all, some 470 groups have been identified. Estimates are made of the costs for a given group, and the median of these estimates used as the basis of reimbursement by the Medicare system. For example, costs for apparently identical treatment of a heart attack were found to range from $1500 to $9000, and a base rate payment of $3100 was determined. Each DRG has a weighting factor based on severity. The weighting factors range from very low (e.g. 0.1309 for false labour) to very high (e.g. 11.9225 for a heart transplant). For most hospitals the average weight is 1.2–1.4 and this average is used as the hospital's 'case mix index' (CMI). Payment is determined by multiplication of the specified DRG weighting factor by the base rate.

As a consequence of DRGs, hospitals with high costs are stimulated to review their procedures in order to reduce costs (previously the opposite applied, because the higher were the costs, the larger was the profit). Opportunities for cost reduction arise in many areas, but particularly in length of hospital stay and ancillary procedures such as sophisticated radiology. Equally the hospital which was already efficient could endeavour to become still more so and thus increase its profit margin; this applies particularly to well-managed, high-throughput surgery (Omenn & Conrad 1984).

The development and implementation of DRGs has only been possible with the advent of the computer. Without computerised billing systems it would have been impossible to ascertain the necessary information on costs. Furthermore, it has been clearly shown that making cost information available to physicians has a favourable effect on both economics and the quality of medical care (Omenn & Conrad 1984). The use of DRGs has proved a powerful and sophisticated concept in health care management and pilot studies are in progress on their use in the UK and other European countries (Sharples 1991). One of the major problems of translation is that Europe uses the ICD-9 system of classification whereas in the US the more detailed ICD-9-CM system is applied (see Chapter 8).

Public-sector management in the UK

Public-sector resource-driven systems suffer from a quite different problem, but this again will be partly solved by the advent of the computer. The problem is that of identifying the actual resources devoted to a given event. Take, for example, a simple appendicectomy for acute appendicitis. Until fairly recently, the managers of a public-sector hospital in the UK would have found it difficult to define the average costs of such a procedure, or even what fraction of their total resources were devoted to the procedure. As a consequence, they would have had no idea whether appendicectomy in the unit was carried out in an efficient or an inefficient manner. However, if information is available and inefficiency can be identified, then action can be taken which frees resources for other purposes. Management of this type is only possible with proper information.

The Griffiths and Korner Reports   An essential part of the use of computers in administration of government-funded medical care will be the promise of management information of the type described above. Indeed, as with demand-led systems, adequate management information can only be obtained through the use of computerised systems.

The will to achieve good public-sector information in the UK has been encapsulated in two well-known reports – Korner and Griffiths – both of which have subsequently been the subject of specific government action. The Korner report consisted of seven documents published between 1982 and 1984; the main purpose was to identify a minimum data set which could be used by all UK health districts in a standardised format. The data include a variety of demographic and administrative items together with diagnoses based on the ICD-9 system. The aim was to describe health care as episodes of contact between the patient and the actual services provided. Central to these, in the hospital sector, is the in-patient admission (the same measurement unit used for DRGs). When a full costing of resources is added to this information ('resource management'), the result should enable a manager to identify the exact costs of an appendicectomy. More important, he or she will know that an identical description will be available for all other units in the UK, and that a direct comparison of 'efficiency' will be possible. In the past, such comparisons have always failed because of different descriptions: hospital X's 'costs' appear to be greater than those of hospital Y, but hospital Y had omitted to include charges for ancillary diagnostic services. These problems are being solved in the UK, albeit slowly, by the introduction of DRGs and equivalents. Methods of describing the relative workloads of hospitals are also being developed under the general heading of 'case mix classification'. Case mix management systems (CMM) collect patient information and assign them to DRGs.

The Griffiths report*, which led to a major reorganisation of management structures in the National Health Service, also reinforced the points made above by mandating that the efficiency of health-care services will be judged by performance indicators. These indicators bring together, in effect, budgeting information with the information garnered by the Korner systems, and have further implicit assumption that the results will actually be used to change a system if it falls short of optimal efficiency.

The influence of computer management systems on clinical data collection

One notable side-effect of the growing cost-consciousness of medicine in both the US and the UK is a dramatic increase in the demand for clinical information by administrators. The information is essential to the proper implementation of DRGs or Korner data sets. Administrative pressure of this type will do more to ensure the rapid installation of patient-oriented information systems than any amount of argument as to the clinical benefits which might accrue. For example, in the first year following the legislation on DRGs in the US, expenditure on hospital computers increased by 20%.

Computers and management forecasting

Computers obviously play a vital role in collecting the information upon which management decision-making can be based. Equally important is the assistance they can give to the actual decision-making by allowing theoretical forward planning, especially of budgets. The decision-making process is greatly helped by the ability of the computer to carry out a series of 'what if' exercises on a matrix of rows and columns (Fig. 2.2). Spreadsheets of this type are widely available on microcomputers but are unusual on larger machines. The best known are '1-2-3' (Lotus) and Quattro (Borland)†. Although these programs only produce what can be

---

* Reviewed in the *British Medical Journal* 287:1391–1394 (1983).
† Reference to applications programs in this book always selects a single familiar example. In reality there are numerous competing spreadsheet packages. Specific packages aimed at Healthcare administration in the UK are available from B-PLAN Software UK Ltd, 11 Whitworth Street, Manchester M1 3GW, UK and Strategic Futures Limited, 8 Mill Pool House, Mill Lane, Godalming GU7 1EY, UK.

| | year | | | | |
	1	2	3	4	5
Budget allocation	78	81	84	87	90
Staff	62	64	66	68	70
Consumables	16	17	18	19	20
	–	–	–	–	–
Cumulative under- or (over-) spending	0	0	0	0	0
Budget allocation	78	81	84	87	90
Staff	47	49	51	53	55
Consumables	20	21	22	23	24
Capital (75/5 years)	15	15	15	15	15
Cumulative under- or (over-) spending	(4)	(8)	(12)	(16)	(20)
Budget allocation	78	81	84	87	90
Staff	47	49	51	53	55
Consumables	16	17	18	19	20
Capital (100/5 years)	20	20	20	20	20
Cumulative under- or (over-) spending	(5)	(10)	(15)	(20)	(25)

Fig. 2.2. Why a spreadsheet can be a very practical management tool. A head of department approaches the unit manager with the suggestion that they could make do with one less staff if given a major item of capital equipment, together with a small increase in the consumables' budget. The manager sets up the forecasts shown in the top and centre panels, which clearly show that the change is not justified on financial grounds. It is then suggested that the consumables' budget would remain the same if a slightly more expensive piece of equipment were purchased. The bottom panel shows that this scenario is even worse financially. This type of exercise, which with current software can be extended to literally hundreds of lines in each direction, represents an enormous advance over the traditional 'intuitive' approach to management which would probably always conclude that machines are cheaper than humans.

performed manually, they do so with such ease and swiftness that they add an extra dimension to the whole process of numerical management.

Among other widely used software tools are project management programs which apply the techniques of critical path analysis and 'program evaluation and review technique' (PERT). These programs deal with a large project as a series of tasks each with a name, timing, cost, personnel involvement and a list of associated jobs which must be completed first. Programs of this type are invaluable to the medical administrator faced with a task such as opening a new clinic, planning seminars, etc.

Major health-care planning activities would today not be possible without computer support. Most large health-care providers have specific groups devoted to computer support for planning, a good example being that set up by the Veterans Administration in the US (Kilpatrick et al. 1988).

Expert systems in medical administration

The topic of expert systems is dealt with in detail in Chapter 5. Here it should be noted that they have administrative as well as diagnostic application. An example is determining eligibility for Medicaid reimbursement in the US. The requirements for this are so detailed and complex that providers often fail to apply for payment with consequent loss of revenue. An expert system has been described which carries out this determination on a microcomputer (MEDELEXS; Sear 1988).

Installing a computer system

The desirability of the various computer applications described in this book cannot be in any doubt. Equally beyond doubt is that their installation can present many problems.*

Where a function is a long-established computer-application – for example, payroll – it is fairly straightforward to purchase and implement an 'off-the-shelf' package which is almost certain to prove satisfactory. However, less well-established applications can present quite formidable difficulties. A notable instance in the UK has been the installation of patient administration systems based on the recommendations of the Korner Report. Several such attempts provoked bitter and even litigious recriminations between health service managers and computer manufacturers.

There are a few simple principles which should be remembered if major surprises and disappointments are to be avoided.

1. There must be a clear institutional commitment to the project. Without this, systems will rarely go beyond the research stage.

2. It is common to underspecify hardware, especially with respect to disk memory capacity and the number of terminals and simultaneous users who can be accommodated. If a complete hospital system is envisaged, it is unlikely that the number of terminals will be less than the total number of beds. Indeed, the most advanced systems involve

---

* Readers are particularly recommended to Broekemeier et al. (1986) and Royce (1987) for a catalogue of woes which may beset a new computer installation; to Lincoln & Aller (1991) for a very detailed review of vendor selection and contracting; and to Warren (1992) for an account of how the Wessex Regional Health Authority in the UK wasted more than £20 million on a region-wide network.

a terminal at every patient 'site' – in-patient bed or out-patient couch. For a major system, an exact specification should be produced which defines the maximum number of transactions per hour and the acceptable response time (typically less than 2 seconds).

3. Underestimation of costs is a very common problem. Software can cost as much or more than hardware, and the costs of staff and staff education associated with a new system may be greater than that of the hardware and software together (especially with micro systems running standard software packages). There is a tendency for software suppliers to underestimate hardware costs and vice versa. The numerous 'minor' items required can reach a quite substantial total (e.g. computer stands, surge protectors, tapes and disks, printer hoods, cables, static mats and printer supplies). Maintenance typically amounts to a recurring annual charge which is 10 per cent or more of the initial capital cost. If possible, there should be a single maintenance contract covering both hardware and software: this avoids the common situation in which one supplier tries to shift responsibility to another.

4. Underestimation of communication requirements is also common; communications can easily represent half or more of the hardware in a system. In most situations the cost of cabling for a terminal (£650; $1000) is greater than that of the terminal itself (£200–£400; $250–$1000), even more so if the terminal is away from the main hospital site. Furthermore, some 50 per cent of terminals are relocated within the first year, and 30 per cent are moved in any subsequent year. This emphasises the need for an extensive and flexible cable infrastructure, installed at the beginning of a project.

5. Every effort should be made to define the purposes and structure of the system in advance.* This sounds almost insultingly obvious but it is extremely difficult to achieve in practice. Good planning should start with the appointment of a task force the function of which is to review current needs and then identify a system which will meet those needs – the procedure referred to as systems analysis (Table 2.4). The group should include representatives from data processing and the specialty involved, but should not exceed five in number. It is wise to accept that even with good planning the initial specification will always fall short of eventual demands, and to make appropriate allowances. This author has never seen a medical system in which the number of terminals did not double between the original plan and the final installation.

---

* It has been postulated that for each hour *not* spent in planning, three to five hours of recovery will be needed.

Table 2.4. The essential questions which must be addressed during the planning process leading up to the installation of a computer system

---

1. What is being done?
2. Who is doing it?
3. Where is it being done?
4. Why are they doing it?
5. When, in the work, or in the working day is it being done?
6. What documents are being put in?
7. What documents are being taken out?
8. What records are being kept?

---

6. For a system of any size (broadly speaking, those costing £50 000 (approx. $770 000) or more a project management structure must be defined (Fig. 2.3) and both the customer and the supplier must appoint at least one person who is available to the project on a full-time or near full-time basis for a minimum period of one year. In the clinical setting an experienced nurse is often the best person to fulfil this role. Failure to do this, especially on the customer side, is a common cause of apparent system failure. An additional advantage of 'dedicated' staff on both sides is to provide a better level of mutual understanding.

7. Although suppliers of computer systems are often much more knowledgeable than the customers, they are not infallible. This is especially the case with major hardware manufacturers, who may make excellent equipment but do not always have the software skills to fit the machine to the application. Similarly, consumers should beware the siren song of many so-called turnkey systems – the complete package of hardware, software, documentation and training. Unless such a package can be clearly seen to be working for the identical purpose on other sites, implementation may demand far more time and effort than is envisaged by either supplier or customer. Some protection against this type of problem can be obtained by the development of in-house expertise in medical informatics.

8. With larger systems managers should be prepared to pay for initial design studies including benchmark analysis to establish the necessary power of the central processor. Leaving this to the supplier as a by-product of bidding for contracts has often proved to be a false economy. Similarly, it should be remembered that the cheapest solution is not necessarily the best (nor is the most expensive), and that a 'pick and mix' approach between the products of different suppliers can be a recipe for disaster unless the user is very experienced and sophisticated.

9. With very large projects increasing use is being made of Computer

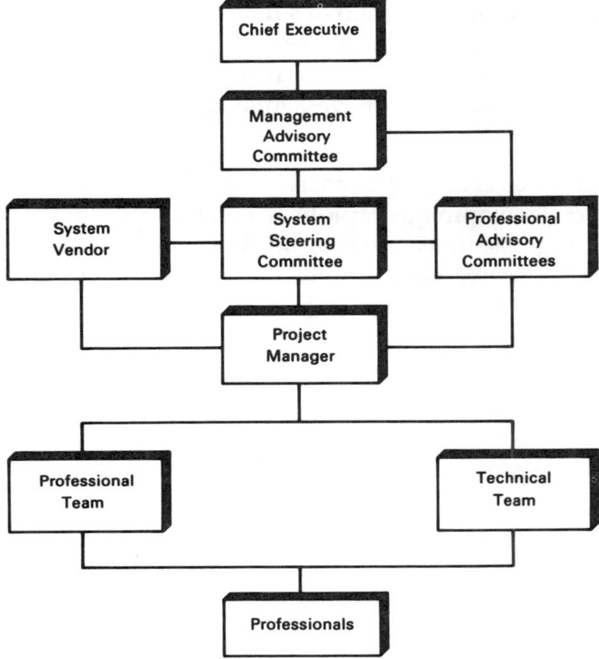

Fig. 2.3. A generalised project management structure for the implementation of a new medical computing system. There are obviously many variations on this, especially in respect of the number of people working in the project team. There are a number of specific programs for project management, e.g. Project Management in a Controlled Environment (PRINCE).

Assisted Software Engineering (CASE), a term which describes automation and integration of the systems analysis and programming steps. In effect CASE is a 'system for developing systems'; CASE renders the whole team less dependent on the skills and whims of the individuals who make up the team.

10. While forward planning is essential, it should not be allowed to become overkill. Benson (1991) has pointed out that a procurement exercise can easily exceed 30 per cent of the total cost of a system. An 'operational requirement' (OR) can extend to over 1000 pages; in the UK, the Department of Health guidelines for suppliers' response has 13 chapters and 53 itemised headings. The result can be a mountain of paperwork which is hardly read by either contracting party.

11. Allowance must be made for training of users; in a clinical setting these may be numerous and of widely differing skills. Allowing staff to practice on model systems is of great value in this respect. Involving potential users at the earliest possible stages of planning and implementation will amply repay any effort involved. Most so-called

opposition to the introduction of a new computer system proves to be a failure of communication between those responsible for installing the system and those (doctors, nurses, etc.) who will use it. This is why it is so important to have actual users on the implementation team.

Finally, it must be recognised that some teething troubles are inevitable with a subject developing as rapidly as computerised information technology. Few organisations, medical or otherwise, are fully equipped to deal with the explosive growth which will occur between now and the end of the century.*

---

* In the UK alone some £500 million will be spent on medical computing in the next 7–10 years. It has been estimated that some 20 per cent of this will be wasted by various forms of system failure due to poor design and implementation.

3

Computers as part of medical equipment

Computers are an essential part of most high-technology equipment used in clinical medicine. Many topics, such as sophisticated laboratory procedures and advanced imaging techniques, have only become possible because of the use of computers.

Introduction

Computers form an integral part of a wide variety of electronic equipment used in both clinical diagnosis and therapy. This is a role which is sometimes less obvious than that of other applications. Many people recognise a 'computer' when it appears as a traditional screen and keyboard, but might not realise that some of the incredibly sophisticated current imaging technology is entirely dependent on computer reduction of quite simple original signals. The great advances in axial tomography have been not in the production and detection of X-rays, but rather in the use of mathematics and hence computation to produce images in a form which was totally unavailable with earlier techniques.

In this chapter the use of computers as part of other machines will be discussed under four general headings: signal analysis, data reduction, laboratory equipment and imaging.

Computers and signal analysis

An important part of clinical diagnosis is the detection and quantitation of signals from various pieces of equipment. A classic example is the measurement of blood-pressure by mercury column sphygmomanometry, which combines auditory signals (the Korotkow sound heard through a stethoscope) with optical signals (the height of the column of mercury relative to a scale). Today, many primary signals from medical equipment are converted into electrical impulses and presented as quantitative information derived from those impulses. The devices which perform this conversion are known as transducers: examples are shown in Table 3.1.

A transducer produces an electrical 'copy' of the primary information. Many traditional devices were based on more or less direct observation of

Table 3.1. Examples of forms of energy which may provide the input signal of a transducer

---

Temperature (e.g. thermometers, thermocouples, liquid crystals, thermography)

Displacement (e.g. strain gauges, induction coils, ultrasound, motion (Doppler ultrasound), force)

Pressure (e.g. occlusive cuffs, tonometry, catheter-tip transducers)

Flow (e.g. electromagnetic flowmeters, ultrasound)

Electrochemical forces (ion-specific, pH and dissolved gas electrodes)

Light (photon detectors)

Bioelectric potentials (e.g. electrocardiographs, electroencephalographs, electro-myographs)

---

the fluctuating electric current so generated, the so-called analog signal. However, with the advent of the computer it is now usual for the signal to be converted from analog into digital form, i.e. from a continuous wave to a list of numbers. The state of the electrical signal is sampled at regular intervals and the findings recorded as voltage and time (see Fig. 3.1) – a process known as analog-to-digital conversion. The great advantage is that the digested information can readily be subjected to further mathematical manipulation.

Automated analysis of a digital signal

The array of numbers produced by an analog-to-digital converter can be processed in two ways: either as a fairly straightforward analysis of the variation of voltage over the course of time (time domain analysis) or as a more complex analysis of the overall pattern of voltage changes (frequency domain analysis).

Time domain analysis

The simplest example of time domain analysis is the search for single discrete events as judged by the signal passing through a predetermined threshold of amplitude: this would be the basis of counting a pulse-rate. Another simple form of on-line analysis is digital filtration to remove all signals which lie outside predetermined thresholds. Other analytical techniques of this type include:

1. Detection of deviation from a baseline: a change in slope indicates the onset of a signal.
2. Turns analysis: detecting reversals of potential.
3. Zero crossing: looking for the point at which the slope of a wave becomes zero in order to detect a peak.

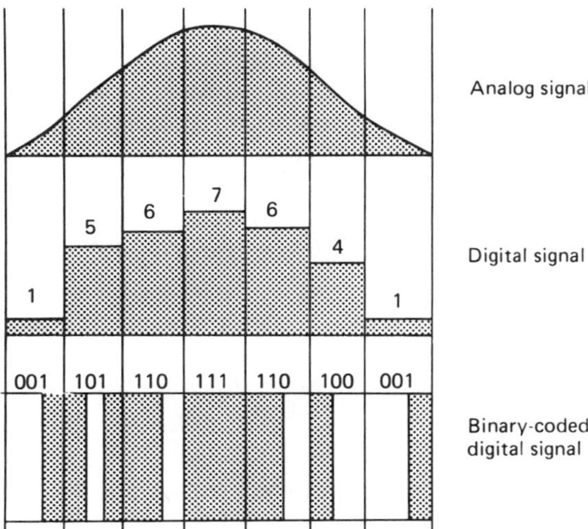

Fig. 3.1. The principle of analog to digital conversion (ADC). The analog waveform (top panel) is sampled at regular intervals (centre panel) and the amplitude at each point converted into binary form (bottom panel). This diagram has been much simplified by the use of a 3-bit system which allows description of only eight different amplitudes (voltages). In reality many more bits would be used to give a much more accurate description. For example, 8 bits would allow 256 different levels (2^8); in a total range of 10 volts, 5 volts would then be represented by the number 128. Medical equipment often requires even higher resolution over a very wide range, and for this purpose 20-bit or even 24-bit ADCs are used. Similarly, in order to obtain an accurate picture of a complex waveform the sampling frequency would have to be greater than that shown here. The limit on this for real-time applications is determined by the clockspeed of the processor and the type of program being run (assembly language routines are much more efficient than interpreted BASIC).

4. Signal averaging: this is used to extract signals from background noise. The amplitude of the wave is summed at intervals: the noise (random + and −) will cancel out while the real signal is enhanced and thus can be reliably identified.

Frequency domain analysis

The standard mathematical process for describing a regular waveform is known as Fourier analysis. The Fourier transform (FT) is based on the fact that any waveform, however complex, can be modelled by a combination of sine and cosine waves. The FT is like a mathematical prism which breaks down a waveform into its sinusoidal components (Fig. 3.2). Each of these waves is a harmonic of the fundamental frequency (i.e. 2, 3, 4, etc., times this frequency); the set of such harmonics constitutes the

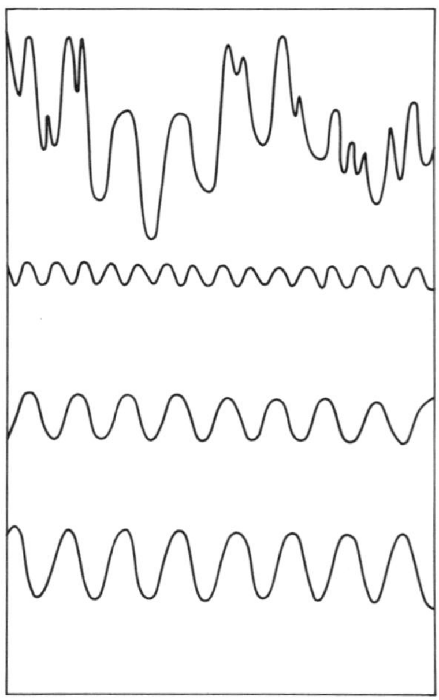

Fig. 3.2. The principle of the Fourier transform. Addition of the lower three sine waves produces the upper, random appearing waveform. The Fourier transform reverses this process, taking the composite waveform and extracting its component sine waves.

frequency spectrum of the original signal, in other words, a digital expression of a complex wave function. A simple waveform such as arterial pressure can be modelled by as few as 10 harmonics; a more complicated waveform such as the QRS complex of an ECG takes 30–60 harmonics. Using this approach a computer can determine the frequency spectrum from a digitised signal. The process uses a mathematical algorithm developed by Cooley and Tukey (1967) which greatly reduces the number of computations required and is therefore called the fast Fourier transform.

With the sort of signal sampling described above, there is a fairly obvious relationship between the power of the computer and the quality of the result. Thus, the greater the frequency of sampling (i.e. speed), the more accurate will be the representation of the waveform.* When computer equipment was slow and of limited availability, it was usual to record the analog signal on magnetic tape for later analysis. Today, many of the same functions can be served by built-in real-time computational facilities – a feature, for example, of many current electrocardiographs.

---

* As a general rule the sampling rate should be double the highest frequency component in a signal (the so-called Nyqvist frequency). Thus, for electrocardiography, a frequency of 500 Hz is recommended.

Connecting medical devices to computers

Most medical devices are now provided with a data output port (RS-232) for connection to a computer. This port is usually of the simple send-only type with two wires: 'data out' and 'ground'. Most computers also have an RS-232 port, making connection an apparently straightforward task. However, communication problems frequently arise necessitating special interfacing hardware and software. It is likely that these problems will be solved with the introduction of the standardised IEE P1073 Medical Information Bus.

Computers and data reduction from medical equipment

Once the primary electric signal has been refined, the next step is to assemble the refined data into a clinically meaningful form. There are many practical examples of this process of which the most familiar is analysis of an ECG. The actual process of analysis may vary from the simple to the very complex. A simple example is counting events and dividing them by the time base in order to yield a rate. A more complex approach is 'template' or pattern matching, where the pattern may be theoretical or real. Algorithms are used to determine the probability that an observed waveform is the same as that of a template, and the use of multiple templates then permits the classification of data into predetermined groups (Fig. 3.3)

Analysis can be performed off-line or on-line. With the 'off-line' approach the signals are recorded (in analog or digital form) onto magnetic tape for later analysis by computer; the tape can be played back at a fraction of the original recording speed to allow time for complex mathematical analysis. With the on-line approach the signals are examined immediately without prior storage or transfer.

Examples of the use of computers for analysis of data from equipment directly interfaced to the patient are shown in Table 3.2. With the continuing reduction in processor costs there is a tendency for all diag-

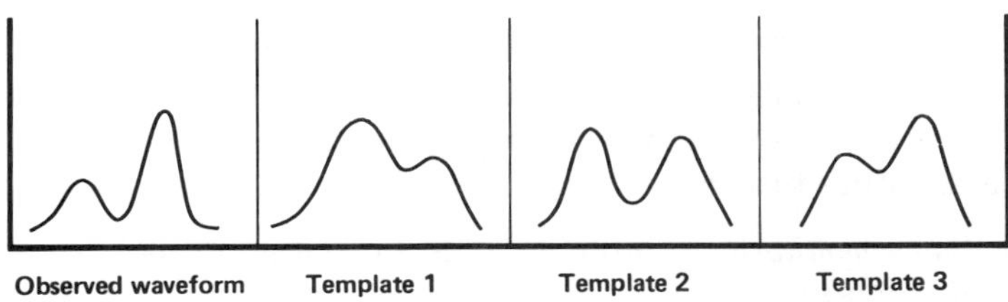

Fig. 3.3. Pattern or 'template' analysis. The observed waveform shown on the left is compared with the three predetermined templates shown on the right. Template 3 is the closest match and the observed pattern would therefore be categorised under this heading.

Table 3.2. Examples of the use of computers for analysis of data from equipment directly interfaced to the patient

Procedure	Reference
Electrocardiography (ECG)	
Foetal cardiotocography (CTG)	Stigsby et al. (1986); Divon & Boucher (1990)
Electroencephalography (EEG)	Simons & Pronk (1983); American Psychiatric Association Task Force (1991)
Intensive care monitoring devices (urimeters, oximeters etc.)	
Urethrocystography	van Mastrigt & Kranse 1993

nostic equipment to incorporate its own computer and therefore to provide on-line analysis.

Despite the increasing power and sophistication of computerised signal analysis it must not be forgotten that the eye and brain are particularly well-suited for rapid pattern recognition. A human can pick out a QRS complex even when there is a steeply changing baseline, and can readily exclude artefacts which might bring a machine to a complete halt. Many current systems use a human to 'clean' the data on a qualitative basis before it is presented to the computer to perform the tasks to which it is best suited.

Computers and electrocardiography

Computers play a particularly important role in electrocardiography (Bessette & Nguyen 1989).* At the machine level the computer permits automatic lead checking, baseline correction, on-line calculations, simultaneous acquisition of data from 12 different leads, noise reduction (using redundant information in simultaneous leads), storage on magnetic media, and transmission for remote processing. Current analysis programs can readily distinguish P, QRS, ST, T and U waves, and can also measure the R-R, PR, QRS and ST intervals. At the diagnostic level there are now several systems for interpretation of the 12-lead electrocardiograph, the best-known being those produced by Hewlett Packard and Marquette. Other functions allowed by the computer include:

1. *Arrhythmia monitoring*: automatic detection of abnormal rate patterns with appropriate alarm functions. For example, atrioventricular block can be diagnosed by identification of a PR interval greater than 200 milliseconds.

---

* This topic has been reviewed in detail in an issue of *Methods of Information in Medicine* (Vol. 29, No. 4, 1990).

2. *Ambulatory recording*: analysis of a 24-hour record at 60–360 times real time, with plots of ST segment deviation against time to document myocardial ischaemia.
3. *Exercise testing*: automatic control of a treadmill according to pre-determined criteria.
4. *Comparison of current readings with previous recordings on disk.*

Comparisons of computer-assisted ECG interpretation (Marquette) with that of visual inspection by clinicians have shown a high level of correlation with no systematic bias (Mulcahy et al. 1986a). A 'normal' report generated by the computer can be relied upon in most cases (Mulcahy et al, 1986b). But there is also much discussion on the relative roles of the machine and the clinician in interpreting ECG data. Macfarlane (1990) has concluded that 'the computer … provides a second opinion which can be accepted or rejected by a physician depending on his own experience'. Automated ST segment monitoring to detect intra-operative ischaemia can only be interpreted in the context of the total clinical picture (Muller & Barash 1993). Another current problem is that of standardisation: data acquired by an ECG system cannot usually be interpreted by another system. This problem is being addressed by a number of international organisations (Willems et al. 1990, 1991).

Computers in the pathology laboratory

The laboratory is the one area of a hospital, other than finance, in which computers have been used for 10 years or more. The practice of two of the major diagnostic subspecialties – haematology and clinical chemistry – consists mainly of the handling of numbers in a highly structured form and is thus ideally suited to computer assistance.

In contrast to most branches of clinical medicine the use of computers in the laboratory is likely to yield cost-savings – not because of a reduction in staff or other resources, but because more work can be accomplished within the same facilities.

Computers have two main functions in the laboratory: control of the electromechanical function of equipment; and the processing of analytic and clinical data. Only the latter will be considered here.

Analysis of signals from laboratory equipment

Most of the automated equipment in haematology and clinical chemistry is centred around optical transducers such as cell counters, spectrophotometers and radiation counters. The use of computers in analysing the electrical signals from transducers has already been described. Rather more specific to this field of application is the use of computers for the calculation of results from the raw data provided by the initial signal analysis.

Some of this calculation is straightforward arithmetic. In the first instance data are corrected for interference or for blank activity. Second, a derived value is calculated. For example an optical cell counter will enumerate the number of cells passing the detector over a given period of time, and match this with the flow-rate to present the result as a concentration. The detector might also measure the size of each cell (the 'mean corpuscular volume') and calculate the results as a mean and as a variation around that mean. At a rather more sophisticated level the machine may be required to carry out some form of calibration, in other words, to read the result from a sample (the 'standard') with a known concentration of the target material, and then compare the unknown with this result in order to estimate the value of the unknown. This calculation is simple if, as with many enzymes, there is a linear relationship between the concentration and the signal: double the signal means double the level.* Rather more complex is the situation in which there is a non-linear relationship between the concentration and the signal. The best example of this is immunoassay (especially radioimmunoassay) where the complex nature of the dose–response curve is such that a series of standards have to be used (the standard curve). The curve can then be analysed mathematically and the derived equation used for calculation of the results of unknowns. This is an ideal task for a computer (see Chard, 1990b).

Information handling in the medical laboratory

In addition to the analysis of results, computers have other major roles in medical laboratory practice. Most well-equipped units will now register the details of samples in a computer database as soon as the specimen is received, together with the results as these become available. This database can then be used for the following purposes:

1. Preparation of work lists (i.e. from a multiplicity of samples, selecting and listing those for a given test).
2. Preparation of labels and printed forms for each sample with a corresponding reduction of transcription errors and staff time. The labels may incorporate machine-readable information which can be presented directly to an analyser.
3. Acceptance of result and printing of the final report. The avoidance of manual transcription from machine to report not only imposes accuracy, but also represents a massive saving of staff time.
4. 'Flagging' of abnormal values.
5. Acting as the database for the calculation of various quality control parameters.

---

* Given the current hardware, the fact that the relation may be log-linear does not add significantly to the complexity of this operation.

6. Acting as a convenient and rapidly searchable file for telephone and other enquiries.
7. Preparation of invoices and accounts as part of a billing system.
8. Linking up with patient files in other hospital-based systems, thus making results available to wards and clinics via on-line VDUs. It is highly desirable that the laboratory system should be directly linked to the hospital's patient information system, thus avoiding the need for re-entry of data. In some units the clinical request is initiated via a terminal in the ward or clinic.

Computer assistance for laboratory diagnosis

A computer can assemble and analyse groups of results from an individual patient and thus present a cumulative report. Furthermore, it can provide diagnostic and management advice on the basis of such reports. Examples are shown in Table 3.3 and Fig. 3.4. Computers can be used to suggest the most appropriate tests in a given situation and also to advise on the costs of tests: this can lead to a substantial reduction in test ordering (Tierney et al. 1988, 1990; Peters & Broughton 1993).

Computers and medical imaging

Imaging is one area of diagnostic medicine which could no longer be practised without computers (Arenson et al. 1990). Imaging techniques range from the in vivo procedures of the radiology department (X-rays, ultrasound, nuclear magnetic resonance, nuclear medicine) to the traditional optical images of histology and cytology. Some simple optical images, such as those viewed through endoscopes, are also being replaced by images generated by electronic means – the charge-coupled device (CCD) camera. All of these images can be digitised and presented on a computer screen.

Table 3.3. Examples of the use of computers for diagnostic interpretation of laboratory data. This has also been the subject of several reviews (Winkel 1989; Connelly & Bennett 1991)

Application	Reference
Collation of serial blood glucose levels in diabetics	Smith et al. 1985
Analysis of lipid profiles with estimates of cardiovascular risk	Bachorik 1987
Estimation of risk of Down syndrome based on biochemical tests	Wald et al. 1988
Calculating antimicrobial therapy based on culture results	Heizmann et al. 1988

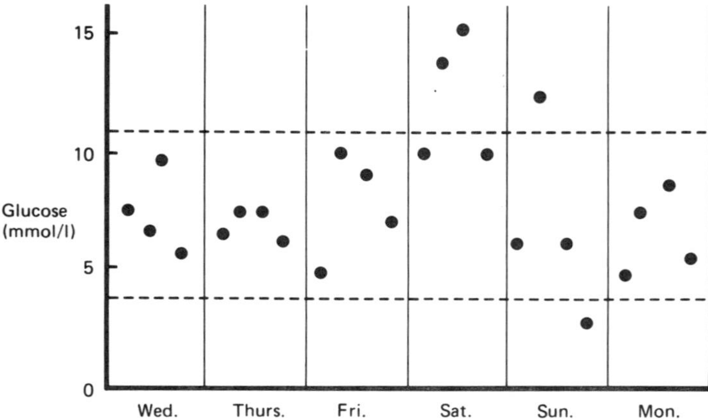

Fig. 3.4. A computer summary as an aid to the management of diabetes. Serial values of blood glucose are determined by the patient using a simple portable reflectance meter, which also stores the results. At the clinic these findings are analysed by a small computer to generate a summary: this clearly shows that control was poor at the weekend and that special attention needs to be focused on this period. (Modified from Smith et al. 1985.)

There is still no more accurate representation of a two-dimensional cross-section of the body than that provided by an X-ray film; nor can any CCD device produce an image equal to that of optical systems coupled to a photographic film. The disadvantage of the simple film, however, is that information is two-dimensional and that it is for all practical purposes 'frozen' in the form in which it is originally produced. The great potential of the computer is that it allows manipulation of images to yield information which would not be accessible by simple visual inspection of traditional media – in effect, the computer can 'see' more than the human eye. Other advantages of the digital, computer-readable image include the potential for a reduction of exposure of patients and staff to X-rays and other forms of radiation, and the ability to store images in a form in which they can be readily and swiftly transmitted to a variety of sites. Currently, some 25 per cent of radiological examinations are digital in origin. It is predicted that when this figure passes 50 per cent there will be a rapid total conversion to digital imaging systems.

The technology of computer imaging: digital imaging processing

Any image can be described as a matrix of small squares (pixels), each containing a shade of grey or a colour. Provided these elements are small enough they blend to form a smooth picture. The imaging sensor can be of many different types (Table 3.4). Some equipment produces a digitized image directly. For computer processing of a standard film the analog

Table 3.4. Examples of imaging systems which may use digital techniques

---

Classical radiography
Computerised axial tomography (CAT)
Nuclear medicine
Contrast radiography
Nuclear magnetic resonance (NMR)
Ultrasound
Thermography
Cytology and histology

---

signal from each element of the original image is converted electronically into a digital signal which describes its intensity and/or colour.

The digital signals are presented as a graphic display. There are three hardware components to this display:

1. A frame buffer, which is usually a RAM chip which stores the image as the matrix of digital values.
2. A display controller, which reads each byte from the frame buffer and passes it to the display device (with a 'refresh' rate of at least 60 times per second to avoid flicker). The display controller or image processor may be a very powerful computer which serves to manipulate as well as simply present the image.
3. A display device, most commonly a cathode ray tube (CRT).

The range of shades and colours will depend upon the number of binary bits available to describe a given point. A 1-bit system can only yield two levels ('0' or '1' equivalent to 'black' or 'white'). Some earlier imaging systems were of this type, but clearly the resolution was very poor: in an X-ray film, for example, it would permit only the identification of the most radio-opaque areas such as bones. Resolution of different structures is much enhanced if each point can be described by several binary bits: 2 bits would yield four intensities, 3 bits would yield eight intensities, etc. A typical television monitor can display 6 bits (64 levels – the maximum which the human eye can distinguish). This is the underlying principle of grey-scale imaging which, if sufficient bits are available, can yield a range of intensities which appears to the human eye as a smooth continuum from black to white. In a colour display each pixel represents a triad of red, green and blue dots and a minimum of 3 bits per pixel is therefore required.

The greater the number of points (pixels) examined, the higher the quality of the image. Up to a density of 128×128 pixels the human eye at a typical viewing distance can see the individual boundaries: this 'pixel clutter' interferes with overall perception of the picture, and for a satis-

Table 3.5. Typical image densities for various imaging techniques. (See Arenson et al. 1990 for a detailed review of this topic)

Imaging technique	Pixels	Typical digital image density	
		Contrast bits	Total kilobytes approx
Nuclear medicine	128 × 128	8	17.4
Ultrasound scan	512 × 512	6	263
CT image	320 × 512*	10 or 12	162/412
Nuclear magnetic resonance	512 × 512	10	526
Radiography	2000 × 2000†	8	4000

* CT images are displayed as a circle and the number of pixels refers to the diameter.
† This is the resolution preferred by radiologists.
The total memory required (kilobytes) includes a provision of 1 kilobyte for header information. Because memory is organised as bytes (8 bits), a 10-bit or 12-bit contrast requires 2 bytes (16 bits) per pixel. A medium-resolution computer screen can resolve 320 × 200 pixels; a standard television monitor can resolve 512 × 512 pixels; high quality systems can resolve 1024 × 1024 pixels; 2000 × 2000 pixel monitors are rare and expensive.

factory image a density of 512 × 512 pixels or greater is required. The information density of a digital image varies greatly according to the technique involved, ranging from the modest requirements of a nuclear medicine image to the very heavy demands of a standard radiograph (Table 3.5).

Presentation of images

The existence of images in digitised form offers great flexibility in the manner of presentation (O'Connell 1988; Smith 1988). However, radiologists continue to prefer the traditional black-and-white image over colour. This is justified by the fact that most images are a two-dimensional map of a single parameter – light intensity or brightness. The human eye can make excellent grey-scale discrimination and simple grey-scale is a perfectly adequate way to display the fluctuations of brightness. The main use of colour is for the dynamic images of nuclear medicine and Doppler flow studies. Radiologists also still prefer hard copy over video display for static images.

Using computers to improve image quality

There are a number of ways in which the computer can improve the basic quality of a digitised image:

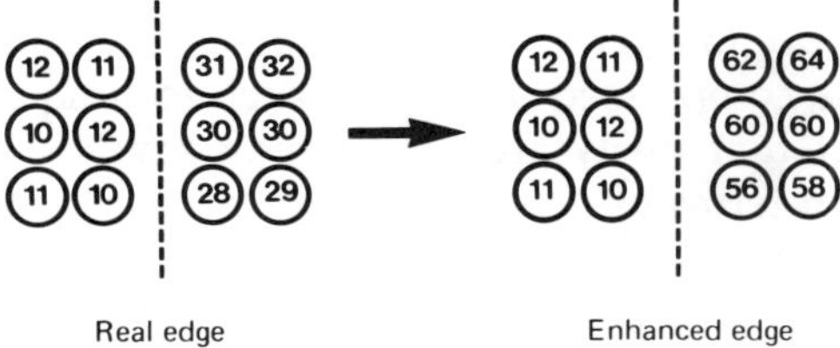

Real edge   Enhanced edge

Fig. 3.5. Computer enhancement of an image. The computer detects the relatively small transitions in intensities between adjacent pixels at an edge, and multiplies those on one side to sharpen the image of the edge.

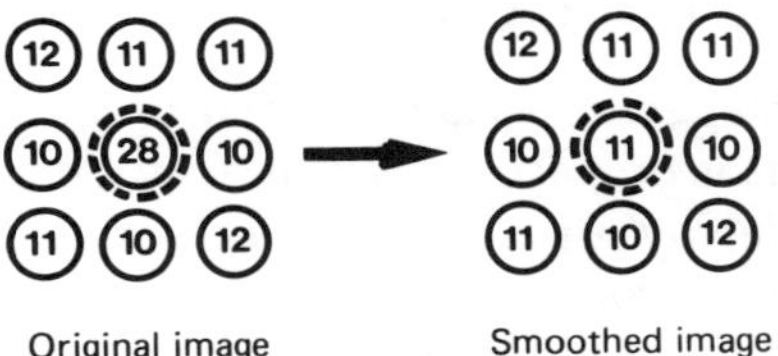

Original image   Smoothed image

Fig 3.6. Computer noise reduction of an image. The computer notes that the central pixel is out of line with the surrounding pixels and adjusts it accordingly.

1. *Enhancement.* A blurred or weak image can often be improved by examining the difference between adjacent pixels. If this difference exceeds a certain threshold, implying that the pixel is part of an edge, then the intensity is automatically increased (Fig. 3.5). Contrast can also be increased by stretching a narrow range of grey levels in a low-contrast image proportionally over a larger range (256 levels). This can reveal features which would not otherwise be apparent. Enhancement has both advantages and disadvantages: thus in chest radiographs it may improve diagnosis of nodules but it also degrades the perception of interstitial disease.

2. *Noise reduction.* This is almost the opposite of enhancement. Small differences between adjacent pixels, which are likely to be due to random noise, are automatically 'smoothed' (Fig. 3.6).

3. *Restoration.* This is the specific removal of non-random noise from images.

4. *Subtraction.* This process is widely used in nuclear medicine, for example, in the localisation of tumours with ^{111}Indium-labelled monoclonal antibodies (MAb). An image which mimics background activity is compared with the MAb image and the final image is made up from the significant differences between the two (Liehn et al. 1987).

5. *Compression.* The very heavy data handling requirements for storage and transmission of medical images make it desirable to 'compress' the data by eliminating redundant parts. There are various techniques for doing this and their performance is compared by the compression

ratio: the storage required for the original image divided by the storage required for the compressed data. One such technique takes advantage of the fact that many areas of a radiograph are more or less homogeneous in terms of density and can be translated into a single number and a set of coordinates. Compression can be particularly useful with serial images for real-time applications, in which only the differences need be recorded. The most recent compression algorithms are capable of reducing a 4 megabyte image to only 0.2 megabyte. More important, relatively inexpensive (c. $500) hardware is now available for compressing images at rates of over 10 million pixels per second (e.g. Microsystems C-Cube).

Manipulation of images, especially in real time, demands substantial computer power. This is one application of so-called parallel processing, and in particular of 'array' or 'vector' processors – a combination of as many as 256 individual processors which execute the same instructions on each clock cycle but on different data originating from the private memory of each processor.

Computed radiography

An alternative to the classic X-ray film is an imaging plate. This has an X-ray sensitive coating which stores the latent image. The plate is scanned with a laser, the emitted radiation is collected by a lens/photo-multiplier combination, and the results are digitised and stored. The advantages of the imaging plate are such that it may replace film in the future (Huang 1987).

Computerised axial tomography (CAT-scans)

A conventional radiograph converts a three-dimensional object into a two-dimensional image. Substantial detail is lost because of the super-imposition of structures. Measurement of X-ray transmission at different angles through a structure (tomography) permits calculation of a three-dimensional matrix of densities. The digital grey-scale values of these densities (the so-called Hounsfield numbers) can be used to construct an image in the form of a two-dimensional slice through the object. This is the principle of computerised axial tomography (the CAT scan) (for which Cormack and Hounsfield received the Nobel Prize in 1979). The computer is an essential part of this process because of the vast number of computations required. A progressive increase in the power of the computer together with advances in source and detector design have reduced the time for a scan from minutes to seconds. The most recent computational development is the production of three-dimensional images.

Picture archiving and communication systems (PACS)

This is the term now generally used for electronic storage and recall of digitised images (reviewed by Schmiedl & Rowberg 1990; Kiuru et al. 1991). (The term Image Management and Communication (IMAC) is also used.) Though obviously desirable, there are important constraints to this technology. The demands on hardware and software are heavy (Hindel 1990). A single picture may require 1 or more megabytes of memory, and for rapid access only high capacity digital optical disks can be used.* Thus it has been estimated that the radiology department of a 1000-bed hospital would generate some 10^{12} bits (1 terabit) of image per year. Real-time images present an even greater problem. The collection of $512 \times 512 \times 8$ bit images at 30 frames per second exceeds the data transfer rates of conventional magnetic disks (1.6 megabytes per second); systems have been described which involve five or more disks working in parallel.

Other constraints are finance and the lack of agreed standards for archiving, for access, for display and processing, and for the user interface. However, it will inevitably happen if only to solve the problem of the 'lost film'; in many units the loss rate is as high as 30 per cent of all images. It has been claimed that the cost-savings to both physicians and patients of a system which guarantees availability could easily repay the cost of the computer installation.

Distribution of computerised images

One of the major advantages of holding an image in a digital computer-readable form is that it can be easily and speedily transmitted to a variety of sites by currently available communication technology. This represents an immense advance over the present situation in which, for example, there is usually only a single set of X-ray films for a given patient and these films are very often not available at the time and place required.

Transmission of complex images requires comparatively high transmission speeds. Within a specialist unit or hospital this will probably be achieved by local area networks using fibre optic links; a 10 megabit image can be transmitted in this way in 5–10 milliseconds. For longer distances use is sometimes made of slow scan television (SSTV), a device which will transmit still video images over ordinary telephone lines. This type of communication has proved particularly useful for transmission of X-ray and other images from remote sites (e.g. ships, research stations, oil drilling platforms) where specialist consultation is not available (Gitlin 1986). However, transmission is slow and quality is usually degraded.

---

* Current optical disks have storage capacity of 1–3 Gbytes and can transfer data at 2–5 Mbits per second. Tapes have much greater capacity but access is very slow.

Newer techniques (image compression; high definition television (HDTV)) have the potential to greatly enhance both the quality and rate of transmission. Though expensive, it has been estimated that the savings from 'telemedicine' might be up to $1500 for every patient who does not have to be transported to an acute-care hospital (*Time Magazine*, May 18 1992, p. 60).

Three-dimensional imaging

The two-dimensional images of traditional techniques can be combined, as a series of parallel slices, to generate a three-dimensional image of a structure. This is an approach which is now much used by industry as 'computer-assisted design' (CAD) and 'computer-assisted manufacturing' (CAM). At one time this required very powerful equipment facilities but sophisticated systems are now available on microcomputers. There is also a move away from geometry-based systems, which build models from the edges detected on a 2D slice, towards voxel-based rendering in which every point is represented directly.

Image workstations

The image work station is a new concept in image evaluation. The work station is a powerful independent computer (or even a microcomputer; Wallin 1993) with a high resolution screen which is used to display and manipulate pictorial information in digital form. This has revolutionised some imaging techniques such as coronary angiography, allowing not just identification of a stricture, but also the exact pattern of the stricture and its effect on myocardial perfusion.

The tools provided by the medical imaging workstation should include (Ratib & Huang 1991):

1. *Image display and formatting*: display in separate screen windows that can be moved and resized.
2. *Dynamic display.* The user can browse through images in a continuous movie mode.
3. *Intensity and contrast adjustment.* The user can choose between different functions and pseudo-colour tables.
4. *Annotations.* Annotations can be added manually.
5. *Filters for image smoothing and enhancement.*
6. *Isocontours.* An isocontouring algorithm for drawing intensity contours at selected levels.
7. *Adaptive histogram equalization*: contrast enhancement which adjusts image so that it uses the available grey levels.
8. *Morphologic measurements.*

9. *Regions of interest.* Circular, elliptical and rectangular regions and irregular polygons can be outlined.
10. *Cross-sectional histograms.* The density profile of a cross-sectional line can be displayed and analysed.
11. *Image combinations*: addition, subtraction, multiplication, and division of two images.

Automatic interpretation of images

Some simple analytical processes, such as looking for small changes in otherwise identical serial images, can be fairly readily achieved with current technology; the process is referred to as registration. An example is the image subtraction techniques used in nuclear medicine. Some degree of pattern recognition is also possible provided the objects examined are simple and repetitive (e.g. automated cytology of blood cells). The understanding of complex images is a branch of artificial intelligence, and especially of neural networks (Lehky & Sejnowski 1988; Lo et al. 1993). Automatic interpretation of images in the sense that a machine can replace or even supplement an experienced radiologist or radiographer is unlikely to come about in this century (Gell 1993). However, it is likely that some degree of machine assistance will be provided for repetitive, tedious work such as scanning for lung nodules (Lo et al. 1993) or assessing texture in tissues such as the placenta (Burger et al. 1987), or the scanning of neuroimages (Banks et al. 1987).

Computers and microscope images

At the present time computers have had less impact on the optical images of histopathology and cytology than on those of the radiology department. However, systems for automated microscopic analysis are beginning to emerge. Karyotyping is one example, in which the labour-intensive process of photographing metaphase spreads and cutting and pasting the picture can now be replaced by digital image manipulation. Further enhancements include automatic recognition of chromosomes (Genetiscan, Perspective Systems Inc, 1301 Regents Park Drive, Houston, TX 77058). Another application is computerised semen analysis. Serial microscopic images are made and analysed to identify motile objects, which can then be counted (Pedigo et al. 1989). However, initial enthusiasm (especially commercial) has been tempered by subsequent experience demonstrating that human intervention is still essential and that automated systems may be highly unreliable (Comhaire et al. 1992). Analysis of microscope images is one area in which neural networks may play a role (Dytch & Wied 1990). PCs are also increasingly used to control the microscope stage and to record the position of images.

4

Computers for clinical data collection

The traditional manuscript patient record is slowly being replaced by the computer based medical record (CBMR). The computer record has numerous major advantages and few disadvantages. However, it will only become universal when there is a keyboard and screen installed at every site of clinical encounter.

Introduction

One of the most rapidly growing activities in clinical medicine is the use of computers for the collection, storage and retrieval of patient data* – in effect, replacing pen and paper with electronic media. A powerful stimulus to this has been the availability of the appropriate hardware and software. Another major factor is the increased demands placed on the medical record: this is no longer oriented solely to patient care, but must also serve communication, quality assurance, accounting and documentation for legal purposes. Even though the implementation of computer systems has been less rapid than was predicted ten years ago, it is now apparent that, before the end of this century, virtually everyone will have some sort of computer-based medical record (CBMR).

In any discussion of computerised data collection it is important to distinguish between data collected prospectively and those collected retrospectively. Prospective data are collected by the clinician at the time of actual contact with the patient: in other words, a screen and keyboard supplement or replace the manuscript notes. Retrospective data are collected after completion of a clinical event, often by clerical staff. Most of the recent growth of this subject has centred on retrospective systems. Retrospective systems are typically much less detailed than prospective systems with broad data items such as 'presenting complaint', 'diagnosis, and 'treatment'. Prospective systems, because they replace the manuscript notes, must be more detailed. The present discussion will address mostly prospective systems, though the basic rules of data collection are virtually identical for both types of system.

---

* Some authors make a distinction between 'data' which is the observation of events, and 'information' which is the organisation of data to guide some question or decision.

Collection of clinical data by computer

The logical structure of all data collection in medicine is summarised in Fig. 4.1. A computerised information system follows exactly the same structure: a question is displayed on the computer screen; the response is entered via the keyboard (or other device); the computer evaluates the response to determine whether it is valid or not; finally, the computer makes a decision either to proceed to another question or to present a conclusion.

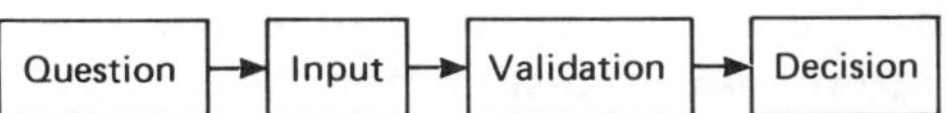

Fig. 4.1. The logical structure of information collection in clinical medicine. Each step begins with a question (which may concern history, physical examination, special investigation, diagnosis or treatment). The response to the question is validated, and leads to a decision – which may be another question or some specific action.

Types of question

Clinical information can be divided into five types: history, physical examination, special investigations, diagnosis and treatment (Table 4.1). History includes all the information which can be obtained by verbal interrogation of the patient or other individuals, together with the information which can be gleaned from written or other records. Physical examination is that non-verbal information which the physician can obtain by the application of his main senses: sight, hearing and touch. Special investigations include all the information which is generated by technology which goes beyond the main senses of the clinician – everything from the simplest blood count to the most complex imaging procedure. The diagnosis is the conclusion reached from the clinical information and treatment is the action resulting from the diagnosis. So far as the computer is concerned all of this information can be collected as

Table 4.1. The five types of clinical information or 'question'

Type of question	Example
History	What is the patient's age?
Physical examination	What is the pulse rate?
Special investigation	What is the haemoglobin concentration?
Diagnosis	What is the diagnosis?
Treatment	What therapeutic action is proposed?

answers to a series of questions, and there is no underlying logical distinction between the different types.

How to design a question

Superficially there should be no difficulty in designing and phrasing a question. However, there are certain rules as to what constitutes a good or a bad question, and the development of a computer questionnaire provides an excellent opportunity to apply these rules.* The first rule is that wherever possible a question should ask for a structured rather than a discursive response (see next Section). The second rule is that it should never be necessary to repeat a question nor should any question appear that is irrelevant in the light of a previous answer. For example, if it has been established that the patient is male, no obstetric or gynaecological questions should be asked. This may sound obvious, but is a common mistake in computer questionnaires which are designed simply by the transcription of a pre-formatted history sheet. The third rule is that the question should always ask for exact data rather than the user's opinion or analysis of those data. Again, this rule may sound very obvious were it not that it is so frequently broken. A prime example is the patient's age, which should always be recorded as the date of birth: the machine can translate this into an age much more rapidly and accurately than can any human (including the patient himself), and will remember to update it after a birthday. Another example is the definition of pathology. A question with the form 'Heart failure: yes or no, and if yes give severity' is likely to be meaningless. The question should be phrased as a sequence of questions each designed to elicit a single fact (e.g. 'Central venous pressure raised: yes or no?'); the computer can then collate these facts to establish 'severity' according to predetermined criteria.

Types of response

A question may be designed to have a discursive or structured response. A discursive response is a piece of free text. For example: 'What is the patient's name?' – 'Chard'; 'Where exactly is the headache?' – 'on the left side'. By contrast, a structured reply only allows selection of one or more predetermined responses. For example: 'Does the patient have a head-ache – yes or no?'; 'Is the headache – 1. on the left 2. on the right 3. at the back 4. at the front 5. all over?'

There are certain pieces of information, such as names and dates, which cannot be prestructured and have to be entered in full. However, as a general rule a structured response should be sought wherever this is

---

* A detailed guide to questionnaire design has been published by Bennett & Ritchie (1975).

possible. The structured response has several important advantages. First, it is convenient and rapid to be able to enter an answer by pressing a single key. Second, it avoids spelling and transcription errors. Third, it provides for the user ready-made definitions of the possible range of responses: an example is shown in Fig. 4.2. Fourth, multiple-choice questions are better than simple 'yes/no' questions for disclosure of factors such as smoking (Mullen et al. 1991). Finally, it provides a very compact piece of code (a single character) for whatever memory device is in use: the equivalent discursive response might typically require a dozen or more characters.

The only disadvantages of structured responses are that they may be difficult to design (which does not mean impossible, merely that they often require time and effort), and that it is sometimes not possible to define every possible option, in which case a discursive 'other' category has to be included in the list. At a research level attempts have been made to design systems which can 'understand' free text by searching for key words and semantic relationships. Such systems are unlikely to be available for routine medical use in the near future. Even if they were available, many would regard them as a retrograde step.

Types of structured response

There are three main types of structured response: (1) a simple 'yes or no'; (2) an exclusive choice from a list, i.e. only one choice can be made and excludes all others (Fig. 4.2 shows an example of this); and (3) a non-exclusive choice from a list (i.e. multiple choices can be made; an example of this is shown in Fig. 4.3). In addition most responses should include 'escape' clauses, in other words, means to respond with a 'don't know' or 'other' or to skip the response altogether. The latter option should only be used sparingly and not as a method for short-circuiting important but tedious information collection.

```
 -------------------------------------------
|                                           |
|  Does the patient smoke:                  |
|                                           |
|  1.   Not at all                          |
|                                           |
|  2.   Up to 10 cigarettes per day         |
|                                           |
|  3.   More than 10 cigarettes per day     |
|                                           |
 -------------------------------------------
```

Fig. 4.2. An example of a question calling for a structured response. Instead of just asking 'Smoking – yes or no?', or 'Smoking – how many?', a list of possibilities is presented which will distinguish heavy smokers from light smokers. These categories could easily be changed or added to if this were believed to be important. In this example the response is 'exclusive', i.e. only one choice is possible.

```
┌───────────────────────────────────────┐
│  What was the endocrine problem:      │
│  1.   Diabetes                         │
│  2.   Thyroid disease                  │
│  3.   Hyperprolactinaemia              │
│  4.   Other                            │
└───────────────────────────────────────┘
```

Fig. 4.3. An example of a structured response with a 'non-exclusive' choice, i.e. more than one of these conditions might be present in the same patient.

Validation of response

One of the key advantages of a computerised clinical information system is the ability to validate each response. This avoids a major problem of traditional manuscript systems which is recording of erroneous or inconsistent material.* The types of validation or error trap incorporated into an interactive questionnaire can be divided into general and specific. General error traps can be further split into transparent and message. Transparent error traps automatically reject any answer that is not one of the options displayed on the screen (Table 4.2). Message error traps are those in which rejection of the answer is associated with a display on the screen explaining the nature of the error and inviting the user to repeat the entry. This type of general trap is aimed at two mistakes, namely making an entry of the wrong length and entering information that is inherently impossible (Table 4.3). It should be noted that general error traps are always absolute. Unlike some of the specific error traps, there is never an option to confirm a response once it has been rejected: it must be repeated in the correct form.

Specific error traps relate to individual questions and are applied after the general validity checks. They are always of the message type and may be absolute or optional, or even a combination. Furthermore, they may be based on information predetermined (Table 4.4) or acquired in a previous section of the questionnaire (Table 4.5). Specific error traps are capable of great flexibility in respect of the limits applied. The staff of a unit can choose for themselves the precise figure at which a response is flagged. In the example shown in Table 4.4 they could define any number less than 20 as the lower limit requiring confirmation of maternal age. The key point is that the presence of limits obviates the more glaring errors that may occur with traditional data retrieval methods.

Some but not all errors can be eliminated by validation procedures. Taking the specific example shown in Table 4.4, if the age of a pregnant

---

* This was also a problem of traditional batch entry computer systems and gave rise to the phrase 'garbage in, garbage out'. All of the validation procedures described here are real-time, that is to say there is an *immediate* feedback on the display unit if the response is not valid.

Table 4.2. Examples of general error traps that are transparent to the user
(i.e. there is no response of any kind if the wrong key is pressed)

Rejection of all keys except Y and N in response to a yes/no question.

Rejection of all letters or symbol keys in response to questions calling for a numeric input (or vice versa).

Rejection of all but a defined range of numbers in response to a choice of a number from a list.

Table 4.3 Examples of general error traps that present a message to the user
(i.e. the answer to the question must be repeated in full)

Rejection of entries of inappropriate length, e.g. a date of more or less than six digits or a time of more or less than four digits.

Rejection of entries that are inherently impossible, e.g. a day greater than 31, a month greater than 12, or a time greater than 24.00.

Table 4.4 Examples of specific error traps on predetermined criteria (the user is invited to confirm the answer or repeat the question)

Maternal age less than 15 or more than 40 years.

More than 10 previous pregnancies, more than six livebirths, or more than three stillbirths, miscarriages or terminations.

Haemoglobin more than 15 g/dl or less than 7 g/dl.

Delivered weight less than 2500 g or more than 4200 g.

These examples are from an obstetric data collection system (Cowan & Chard 1985): a similar set could be developed for any area of clinical medicine. The limits shown here are conditional, i.e. the user is prompted to confirm them. They can be expanded to absolute limits if the range is extended (e.g. maternal age over 60).

Table 4.5. Examples of specific error traps based on information acquired in a previous section of the questionnaire (the user is invited to confirm the answer or repeat the question)

Total number of previous deliveries not equal to livebirths plus stillbirths.

Date of delivery more than one month from expected date of delivery.

Day and time of delivery more than 24 hours from onset of labour.

Complications such as thalassaemia or sickle-cell disease in a patient of an inappropriate ethnic group.

These examples are from an obstetric data collection system (Cowan & Chard 1985) woman is entered at 62 instead of 26 then the error will be flagged. However, if the transposition was from 23 to 32 the response would be accepted.

Validation by secondary questions

A still more sophisticated system of validation is the use of additional questions to ascertain the significance or otherwise of a previous response. A relatively simple example in a general medical history would be the question 'Does the patient have headaches?': a positive response would lead to further questions aimed at identifying (or more usually, excluding) those cases which might be of pathological significance.

The content of a computer questionnaire

The short answer to the question 'What data should be collected?' is 'anything that is useful to the management of an individual patient'. But at a practical level this response is valueless because it begs the question of what is 'useful'. It could equally apply to the medical encounter consisting of 'What is the problem? Headache, doctor. Here is an aspirin' as to the most complex investigation of this particular presenting symptom.

Identifying the content of a computer questionnaire calls for a high level of medical expertise but little technical knowledge of computing. The main contribution of the computer expert is a habit of logical thought and knowledge of systems analysis, both areas in which the physician is often deficient. When it comes to the actual questions, all parties should apply the key criteria of relevance, completeness, accuracy and collectability.

Relevance simply specifies that the questions should have some relation to the patient's condition. The patient with headache will usually be asked about disturbances of hearing or vision, whereas the minutiae of bowel or bladder function can safely be ignored.

Completeness specifies that the question should include everything which might be relevant – for example, that one should not omit to ask about hearing and vision in a case of headache. Not infrequently, however, the demands of relevance and completeness are incompatible. Any second-year medical student should be able to describe pathology which leads to altered bladder function *and* headache, while recognising that the association is rare. Knowing what question to ask and where to stop are the hallmark of the expert clinician. The CBMR must try to emulate this.

Accuracy describes the fact that the answer to a question may deviate substantially from the underlying truth. A notable example of this is a menstrual history: a woman's perception of the amount of her monthly loss, and whether it is normal or abnormal, bears almost no relation to the amount of loss measured by objective techniques.

Collectability specifies what can reasonably be achieved with the available resources (in the case of the history, the patient's or physician's resource is time). An argument could be made for a complete psychiatric evaluation of every case of headache. The reality is that this would be impractical – not to mention unacceptable – in a routine setting. Making the questionnaire 'intelligent' by choosing questions on the basis of previous answers can have a substantial advantage in this respect. Haug et al. (1987) showed that a 'decision-driven' system for the interview of patients with pulmonary disease reduced the number of questions from a possible total of 182 to a mean of 50 per patient, without any loss of diagnostic accuracy.

All of the above discussion has treated a 'question' as an item of clinical history, but precisely the same criteria apply to items of clinical examination and special investigation.

It is important that the content of a questionnaire should be regarded as flexible – in other words, that individual units or physicians should be able to determine, or at least vary, the content of their own database. Such flexibility is readily accommodated by the current technology. It is particularly important at the earlier stages of implementation of a system, when the ability to accommodate individual preferences can have a strong positive effect on the acceptability of a system.

It is sometimes more difficult to determine the content of a retrospective questionnaire than a prospective questionnaire. Although the retrospective record contains many fewer items, there are endless decisions to be made about what to include and not to include. Numerous different demands may be placed upon the system – information for resource management, information for clinical audit. If every possible request is catered for, then a retrospective system can rapidly become almost as detailed as a prospective system.

The initial design and organisation of a questionnaire

The design of a questionnaire is by far the most important of the intellectual exercises involved in the development of a CBMR system. By contrast, the technical aspects of hardware and software are relative straightforward.

Any data collection system involves leading the user through a series of displays and in the design phase of a system the sequence or pathway should be documented by means of procedural flow-charts.

Certain general rules of questionnaire design are worth emphasising:

1. Various categories of staff are usually involved in any system. If some items are entered by clerical staff then it should not be assumed that

the user has a knowledge of medical terms. Simple explanation screens and lists of options can be a great help in this respect.

2. The overall pathway should follow a logical sequence which reflects as closely as possible the non-computer equivalent. Related material should be organised on adjacent screens. This is an aspect of design in which it is essential that the computer expert and the physician work together.

3. Branching to an index should always be possible. This allows immediate access to any screen in the sequence without the need to proceed via all earlier screens.

4. The system must be able to produce summaries which take selected information from a variety of input screens and present it as a coherent unit on a single screen.

5. The system must be able to loop back to any item to allow correction or modification of an entry.

Advantages of computerised data collection

The advantages of computerised data collection are as follows:

1. *Legibility and organisation of records.* Traditional manuscript notes or summaries may be difficult (sometimes impossible) to read and are often poorly organised, each successive contributor using a slightly different order and layout of items. Furthermore, notes tend to be organised according to source, laboratory tests being found in one part of the chart, progress notes in another, and vital signs in yet another part. One of the first things which appeals to the user of a new computer system is the legibility and logical layout of the outputs (screen or printer display).

2. *Standardisation.* Once a system has been agreed and implemented it will always appear in exactly the same form, regardless of when or where it is used. Questions can then be carefully designed so as to produce a standard and meaningful response. For example, the question 'Does the patient drink alcohol?' will produce large numbers of positive responses most of which are of little or no significance. It is obviously much better to categorise the response according to the actual amount consumed, as shown in Fig. 4.4. A screen of this type ensures that the question is always asked in the same way.*

3. *No omissions.* The computer questionnaire provides the user with a meticulous and unavoidable set of 'prompts'. Every formal comparison

---

* In a study on taking an alcohol history, Bernadt et al. (1989) showed that the level of agreement between computer and humans was similar to that between different groups of humans (psychiatrists and psychiatric nurses). For all methods there were occasional wide discrepancies.

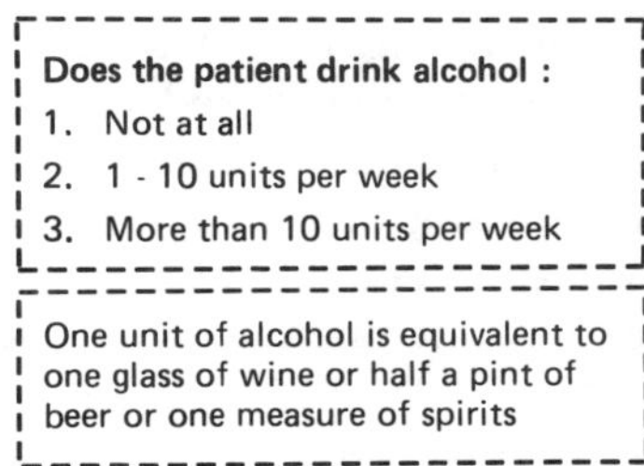

Fig. 4.4. An example of a standardised question. The response must be one of the three categories shown, and there is a 'help' message to ensure that the user understands the meaning of the question.

of structured versus free-form data collection has shown the superiority of the structured approach (reviewed by Erdman et al. 1985), although very few studies have been performed with an acceptable randomised design (Haynes & Walker 1987; Lilford et al. 1992). The number of items included in a computer record is larger and more complete than that of a written record (Jones & Hedley 1986; Quaak et al. 1987). However, completeness is only possible once the clinical problem has been somewhat focused, otherwise large amounts of negative, irrelevant data will be gathered. In real-life a clinician will adapt his or her questioning on the basis of early responses, becoming increasingly detailed as the problem is narrowed down.

4. *Saving on skilled staff.* All computer questionnaires are designed, or at least reviewed, by the most senior and experienced staff in a unit. Consequently the questionnaire will embody the skills of these staff and will closely define the conduct of the clinical encounter. Thereafter the quality of the data collection should be the same regardless of the seniority of the user. For example, it has been shown that a computer-directed algorithm permits triage by minimally trained personnel in an emergency room (Berman et al. 1989). In addition, the use of a computer questionnaire by trainees fulfils an important educational function.

5. *Better collection of sensitive information.* Computer screening elicits more HIV-related factors in the health history of blood donors than does a non-computer approach (Locke et al. 1992).

It can be argued that most of the above advantages would be achieved by a well-structured paper questionnaire. All too often research studies suggest that a CBMR is superior when in fact it is compared to a poorly designed existing system. Comparison of well-designed systems often shows near equivalence (e.g. Lilford et al. 1992). That being said, there are still some advantages which are exclusive to a computerised data collection system:

1. *Widespread availability of information.* Data can be retrieved within seconds at a wide variety of sites linked to the central memory by dedicated lines or telephone lines. This is in sharp contrast to manuscript notes which are available on only one site at a time. The benefits of electronic communication between the hospital and primary care providers has been clearly documented in The Netherlands (Branger et al. 1992).

2. *No loss of information.* Subject only to major electronic breakdown, which is extremely rare, computer notes cannot be lost. This again is in sharp contrast to manuscript notes which, certainly in hospital practice, are very frequently lost.

3. *Electronic supervision.* In many business systems the computer is used to monitor employee performance – for example, the average length of time taken by an airline reservation clerk or a telephone operator to handle a customer. This can produce substantial increases in efficiency, but creates a form of pressure which would not be popular in a health-care environment.

4. *Ancillary checks.* The computer can incorporate ancillary data not available to a pen-and-paper medium, such as the time taken to answer a question (response latency) and the force with which the key is struck.

5. *Convenient document preparation.* Current medical practice involves the preparation of large amounts of ancillary paperwork – investigation requests, notifications to other health-care groups, insurance and reimbursement claims, etc. The word-processing functions of the computer are ideally suited to these operations and it is this aspect of computerised data collection which is often the major initial stimulus to the instalment of a system.

6. *Speed.* Well-organised data can save time. Information can be found faster in a structured computer record than in a manuscript record.

7. *Avoidance of document preparation.* In a truly effective CBMR all the data would be held electronically with no need for a separate set of documents. The feasibility of a paperless clinical record has been demonstrated in obstetrics (Gonzalez & Fox 1989) but it may be some time before this is widely accepted.

8. *Summaries.* A CBMR can help to solve the problem of information overload in a clinical record system. Most systems have facilities to present sets of selected data items from different parts of the record in a single screen or printout. Presentation of a variable number of observations of the same parameter as a flow-sheet can be particularly valuable (time-oriented data), though this is difficult to achieve within some database systems. The most sophisticated systems can automatically analyse complex data and produce elegant graphical displays of high-level concepts (Zegher-Geets et al. 1988).

9. *Medicolegal aspects*. The completeness, availability, and legibility of a computer record may be of great assistance in any subsequent dispute.

10. *Audit*. The whole process of clinical audit creates heavy demands for data retrieval, which can often only be achieved if some sort of computerised database is available. Genuine clinical audits require more detailed and comprehensive data than are generally provided by current retrospective databases (Yudkin & Redman 1990).

Disadvantages of computerised data collection

The major potential reservations about CBMR systems are as follows:

1. *Need for keyboard entry*: This is a major constraint with many clinicians over the age of 30, though it may not apply to future generations. It is one of the commonest reasons for non-acceptance of a system.

2. *Limitation on discursive data*. The use of a computer undoubtedly limits the amount of discursive information which can be recorded. In other words, it is not usually possible to write a 500-word essay on every patient. However, many would regard this as a positive advantage, and applaud the fact that a computer discourages vague entries such as 'Feeling well', 'Better than before' etc. Equally, the recent availability of vast, cheap memory devices somewhat restores the scope for unstructured entries. It would be unfortunate, though, if this detracted from the computer-led trend towards clearly defined, compact data structures.

3. *Loss of doctor–patient relationship*. Virtually every new piece of medical technology is accused of disturbing the doctor–patient relationship. In reality, the replacement of pen and paper with a screen and keyboard should, if anything, enhance the time available for interpersonal communication. This view was confirmed in a study of video recording of computer versus traditional history taking (Brownbridge et al. 1985). Furthermore, virtually every formal study on *patient* acceptance of computer systems has shown a majority in their favour.

4. *Loss of confidentiality*. There will always be concern that personal data held on a computer could be accessed by unauthorised persons or bodies. In reality, computer-held data are generally better protected than manuscript notes (see below).

5. *Hardware and software breakdown*. The implementation of any computer system is usually associated with numerous minor 'glitches', almost always due to software faults or failure of communication systems and networks. These problems are generally solved with a little persistence by the supplier and the user. Nevertheless, it must be recognised that downtime disruption is probably the single greatest cause of user

dissatisfaction with computers. Total hardware failures with current equipment are *very rare*, and the chances of major data loss due to equipment failure can be virtually eliminated by meticulous attention to regular backups. Another problem is that systems can become frustratingly slow when there are multiple users.

6. *Access*. With 'interpretive' clinical data collection systems there is often controversy as to who should have access to the system, and whether access should be confined solely to health-care professionals. There is even interprofessional argument: for example, psychologists have objected to the use of computerised personality data assessment by psychiatrists (see Fowler 1985).

7. *Cost*. Despite claims to the contrary a computerised data collection system will probably always cost more than the manual counterpart. Initial hardware and software costs, amortised over a 5-year period, may be relatively low. However, the extra personnel costs of installing and running a CBMR system may be substantial. For example, batch entry of data into a CBMR system which duplicates a manual system involves additional costs of $5–10 (approx. £3.25–£6.50) per patient encounter. One group reported that 17 per cent of the charge for an office visit could be attributed to the use of COSTAR (Dambro et al. 1988). Though this seems exaggerated, the arguments *for* a CBMR system must be based on improved information handling rather than on cost savings. Under some circumstances, information handling may save resources which would otherwise have to be committed to manual retrieval of data.

8. *Problems of system design*. Even though a 'manual' system is in routine day-to-day use it can be very difficult to emulate with a computer questionnaire. One of the reasons for this is that a manual system is hardly ever perfect, but typically captures only 90 per cent or less of relevant data. By contrast, the computer system must aim at perfection: the acquisition of the final 10 per cent of the data can demand much effort.

9. *Conversions of existing records*. When a system is first implemented most patients will still have traditional manuscript records. The problem may arise of transcribing these to the new system. Even for simple identifying information in a small private practice this can be a herculean task. The usual decision is to let the system run in parallel for a period of time (e.g. 6–12 months) followed by archiving of inactive records.

Examples of CBMRs

CMBRs have been described for virtually every branch of medicine. Some of the more familiar examples of these are shown in Table 4.6. The main

Table 4.6. Examples of well-known computer-based medical record systems (CBMRs) (for a detailed review see Lloyd 1985). The systems listed here are all available to other users. Well-known systems which are not available (e.g. PROMIS from the University of Vermont) have not been included

Name	Site	Features
Computer Stored Ambulatory Record (COSTAR)	Massachussetts General Hospital	One of the earliest programs with highly structured (but off-line) inputs, and outputs available at a variety of community sites (Kerlin 1986)
The Medical Record (TMR)	Duke University	Less flexible than COSTAR, and could only be accessed by one user at a time. However, it is rapid and much used for simple functions (Stead & Hammond 1988).
Summary Time Oriented Record (STOR)	University of California	A network of different computers in different units sharing a common communications protocol (Whiting-O'Keefe et al. 1988)
Regenstrief Medical Information System (RMIS)	Indianapolis	A total hospital information system including comprehensive patient history summaries, alerts, reminders, result monitoring, pharmacy services and billing (McDonald et al. 1988; Martin 1992).
HELP	Salt Lake City	Medical records with extensive decision support (Pryor 1988)
-	Boston	Integrated departmental and laboratory system in three hospitals (Bleich et al. 1989)

With recent advances in hardware and communications technology all of these programs have been updated or replaced by more sophisticated systems. In particular, real-time data entry by multiple simultaneous users is regarded as essential in current practice. It is also important to recognise that most of these systems were devised for ambulatory (out-patient) rather than hospital practice. In addition to the well-known generalised systems, vast numbers of smaller systems dedicated to special topics have been described. Many of these are designed to run on microcomputers using standard database packages (e.g. dBASE, Paradox).

constraint to widespread acceptance and use of many of these published systems is that they will only work on certain types of equipment. For example, COSTAR is written in the MUMPS language which was originally designed for DEC VAX systems and until recently could not be run on IBM machines (Kerlin 1986).

What subjects are suitable for CBMRs?

Some topics are better suited to computerised record keeping than others. For instance, simple single problems such as many of the situations encountered in general practice can be well handled by traditional records. It is also generally accepted that the first encounter with a new patient cannot be computerised because of the enormous potential span of knowledge which is required (Fig. 4.5). Examples of situations which are well-suited to computerised recording include:

1. Conditions which require long-term follow-up, and for which overlooking changes may be hazardous (e.g. chronic renal disease, cancer follow-up).
2. Clinics dedicated to a single or limited number of diseases, with a very routine pattern of data collection (e.g. diabetes, antenatal care).

Improved follow-up as a result of a computer register has been clearly demonstrated in a diabetic clinic (Jones & Hedley 1989).

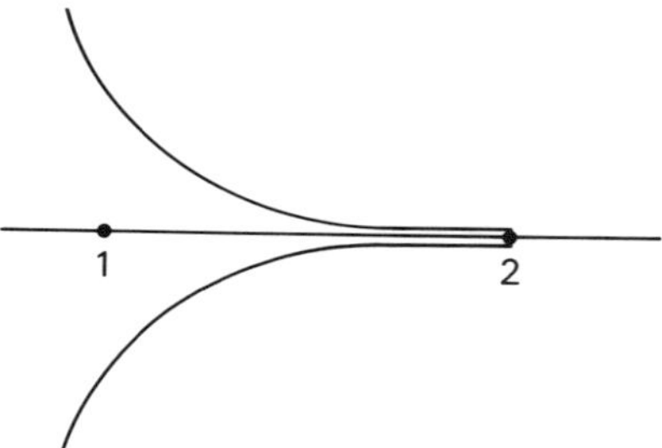

Fig. 4.5. A diagram of the cognitive span required from a clinician during a patient interview. At point 1, where the patient is first seen, the potential range of problems is vast. By point 2, the collection of data has focused the problem to within a narrow domain. Computerised data collection systems are most effective towards point 2 (i.e. once the problem has been focused) (modified from Blois 1984).

Who inputs data into a CBMR?

At the present time most computerised data collection in hospitals is performed by a centralised team of coding clerks. Such staff can easily feel over-worked and remote from clinical activity. A more satisfactory solution is to provide a non-clinical member for each medical team. The ideal solution is for clinicians (doctors, nurses, etc.) to enter data at the point of collection. However, this requires more extensive facilities than are currently available in most institutions.

Self-administered questionnaires

Several computerised questionnaire systems have been designed for direct input of data by the patient. This has obvious advantages in terms of time-saving for skilled staff, and has been particularly applied to the very exhaustive history-taking which may be part of a psychological and psychiatric assessment (Erdman et al. 1985). In addition, patients may reveal personal or sensitive information more readily to a computer than to a physician (Slack & Van Cura 1968; Lucas et al. 1977). This has been demonstrated for items such as alcohol consumption, sexual functioning and suicidal thoughts. The disadvantage of the self-administered questionnaire is that it can only be used where simple and straightforward questions can be formulated and understood with the help of written instructions. Furthermore, there is no opportunity to probe uncertain responses. In a study on a self-administered CBMR for patients with back pain, the error-rate for the machine was higher than that for clinicians (Thomas et al. 1989). However, most of these errors were due to in-adequate question design.

Gathering data from free-text records

Prototype systems exist for extracting structured information from dictated admission summaries (Lin et al. 1992). These systems depend on sophisticated free-text processing (canonical phrase identification). Current efficiency is 90 per cent plus but still not 100 per cent.

Some aspects of computer inputs and outputs

Ergonomic aspects of input and output devices

The optimum input device (or certainly the commonest) is the QWERTY keyboard with associated cursor and special function keys. As a general rule this should be detachable and there should be separate vertical adjustments for the display screen, keyboard and document holders. This allows a comfortable body position for the user – of particular importance in a medical interview where two people may be looking at the screen while only one is making entries. It is interesting to note that keyboard performance (speed and errors) may deteriorate with advancing age (Czaja & Sharit 1993).

Siting of terminals

Most clinical computer terminals are found on a desk in the physician's office or at a nursing station. With falling hardware costs and better network technology there is increasing use of bedside terminals.* These have obvious advantages in terms of immediate availability of data to those directly involved in the case of the patient, and simplification of entry of routine observations. As space is usually limited the physical characteristics of the bedside terminal are important. These include wall-mounting, use of simplified keyboards, and placing the device at standing eye level. Hand-held devices may have a place but usually have a very limited display.

Screen design

It is obvious that the overall appearance of the screen should be helpful and attractive to the user. The design of screen layouts is more of an art than a science, though attempts have been made to provide formal sets of guidelines (Tullis 1983).

To ensure good screen design the following guidelines should be followed:

1. Layout should be standardised so that the same displays and functions always appear in the same areas (see Fig. 4.6).
2. Items should be grouped in a coherent and logical manner (e.g. history and examination should not be mixed in the same area).
3. The layout and order of corresponding data fields should be consistent from one display to the next.
4. The screen should be visually attractive with careful attention to spacing so that the display is concise and uncluttered.
5. The order of items should follow the way people normally read – top to bottom, and left to right.
6. Features such as colours, highlighting, different-sized characters etc. should be used if they are available.
7. Both upper and lower case characters should be used for easy reading.
8. The characters should be readily visible at a distance of 40–80 centimetres.
9. The screen density, i.e. the percentage of the screen occupied by characters, should be as near as possible to the optimum value of approximately 15 per cent. Above 25 per cent there is an increase in time and errors in locating a target.
10. A display should contain ample blank spaces between items.
11. A prompt should be provided for unusually long delays (e.g. 'Please wait while patient record is found').

---

* A number of systems using bedside terminals are reviewed in *MD Computing*, Vol. 4, No 1 (January/February 1988). Costs appear to be $2000–$3000 per bed.

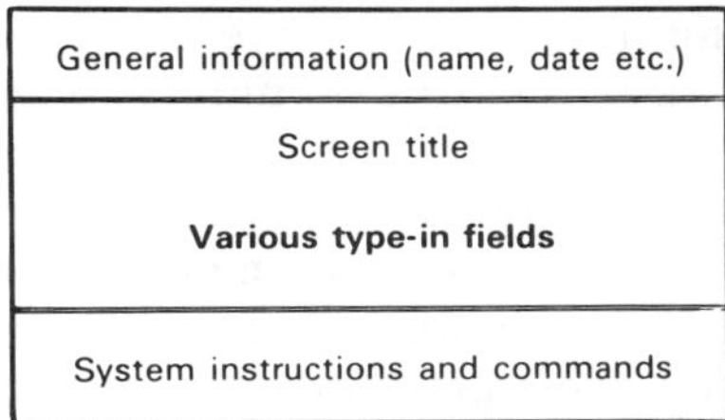

Fig. 4.6. The 'standard' layout of a computer screen for a CBMR system. General information appears in a horizontal panel at the top of the screen, system instructions in a panel at the bottom, and the specific subject matter of the screen in the central area.

12. With the exception of system instructions (Fig. 4.6) the screen should be completely cleared between displays.
13. Scrolling of text should never occur.
14. Blinking or flashing text, although useful for highlighting, should be used sparingly.
15. Although most current screens display light characters on a dark background ('negative polarity'), increasing use should be made of dark on light because this is believed to produce less visual fatigue.
16. Adjustment of brightness and contrast should be possible to allow for the preference of individuals and for differences in lighting conditions.
17. Any feedback responses (prompts, explanations, error messages etc.) should appear on the screen without removing the original display: 'windows' are particularly useful for this purpose. This is an aspect of the basic rule that all instructions needed to operate the system should be incorporated with the system. Separate printed instructions should be confined to how to switch the system on.

Many of the above rules also apply to the preparation of printed documents. It is notable that even with the closest attention to screen design, people still read more slowly from a CRT display than from paper (Gould et al. 1987).

Patient reactions to CBMRs

Every study on patient acceptance of computer systems has shown an almost total majority in favour – undoubtedly helped by the fact that the physician using a computer will give an image of efficiency and advanced practice (e.g. Brownbridge et al. 1985; Rethans et al. 1988).* Strangely, this

---

*To quote John Paulos: 'I'm always amused by commercials for banks which tout ... personalized service; a poorly trained and badly paid cashier saying 'Good morning' and then fouling up your transaction. I'd rather go to a machine which knows me by a code word but on whose ... programs a team of software writers has painstakingly worked for months.'

may not apply to veterinary practice: 'we did not put terminals in examination rooms because ... clients should feel that they are our only concern ...' (Rude 1986). In human practice, most of the criticism about lack of acceptability of computerised systems to patients comes from physicians who themselves feel 'nervous' about the new technology or, worse, that their professional standing is in some way threatened by a machine which emulates their performance. For example, Johnson & Williams (1980) reported that patients were strongly favourable towards computerised personality testing, but that the attitudes of staff ranged from neutral to slightly negative. Brownbridge et al. (1985) concluded that 'patient reactions ... are more affected by which doctor they see than by whether or not the doctor is using a computer'. Furthermore, unfavourable professional attitudes are often based on the use of poorly designed, outdated systems.

The time taken to respond to a question in a CBMR varies between individuals. In one study older women responded more slowly than younger subjects, and women with less formal education took longer to respond (Slack et al. 1988).

Clinicians' reaction to CBMRs

Faced with a good computerised data collection system, most clinicians are positive and enthusiastic. Why then has the introduction of these systems into routine clinical practice been so slow? In the UK, part of the answer may lie in the fact that resources for CBMRs are provided by managers, and this leads to systems which have an administrative rather than a clinical bias. 'These systems ... do little to support patient care and are unpopular with doctors who perceive their function as providing activity data for managers ...' (Lelliott 1994). If genuine clinical informatics is to come of age, then a higher priority will need to be given to the information needs of clinical workers. Administrative data should be a by-product of clinical data, not the reverse.

Speech recognition

Several devices have been described which enable computers to recognise spoken words. Most such devices convert the incoming sound into digital format and then compare this against stored templates. A more advanced process breaks down the sound into phonemes – the smallest recognisable unit of speech – which are then converted into words using a sound-based dictionary. At a still higher level the process examines adjacent sound patterns, word combinations and even grammar.

Speech recognition devices have been classified according to mode of speaking (one word at a time or groups of words at a time), speaker dependence (recognises one speaker (after training) or multiple speakers) and active vocabulary size. There is usually a trade-off among these features. Systems which recognise groups of words from multiple speakers will have a vocabulary of less than 100 words, whereas isolated utterance, speaker-dependent systems may have a vocabulary of up to 1000 words (Akers 1986). To put this in context, it has been estimated that the minimum vocabulary required for automated dictation is 5000 words. The response time for a voice recognition system should be 150 milliseconds or less. Complete speech analysis systems are now available commercially (e.g. CSL Computerised Speech Lab, Key Elemetrics Corp, 12 Maple Avenue, PO Box 2025, Pine Brook, NJ 07058, USA). An example of an automated history-taking system using speaker-independent continuous speech has been described by Johnson and colleagues (1980).

Speech recognition systems are sometimes thought of as expensive and sophisticated toys. However, they have much potential for serious application: for example, control of equipment and data entry when the user's hands and eyes are already busy (the operating room) or when the environment is darkened (an ophthalmology suite). Furthermore, voice-controlled robotic devices have been developed for quadriplegics.

Data collection using portable equipment

Current technology includes powerful microcomputers which will fit in a brief-case or even a pocket. These can be used for data collection at a wide variety of sites not equipped with terminals (e.g. community care). Examples of this type of equipment include the range of hand-held devices produced by Psion (Psion Ltd, Psion House, Harcourt Street, London W1H 1DT, UK) (Green 1986); the Clinicom system in which a hand-held device communicates with a base station by radio frequency (CliniCom Inc, 4720 Walnut Street, Suite 106, Boulder, Colorado 80301, US); and the Telxon systems (Telxon, Old Orchard, High Street, Poole, Dorset BH15 1AE, UK). Systems using a pen and a graphics tablet may have a significant future.

Data protection

It is widely believed that the existence of personal data in electronic form offers the opportunity for various users to obtain this information and, implicitly, to use it to the disadvantage of the individual concerned. Probably the most sensitive area of this type is personal financial information – whether or not a person is a good 'credit risk' – and there are endless horror stories about those who have received a lifelong electronic stigma as a result of one small oversight in credit payment. Other sensitive areas include criminal and political records. With few exceptions (such as sexually transmitted diseases) medical records are rather less sensitive than financial and social topics. A man may well not wish it known that his driving licence has been suspended and that he owes the bank a substantial sum of money, but be quite indifferent to publicity about his broken ankle. Nevertheless, it is generally accepted that every reasonable effort should be made to ensure the confidentiality of medical records, either paper or electronic. 'Reasonable', in this context, must take account of the fact that large numbers of people may quite properly need to access medical records: the aim is to exclude unauthorised users without making life difficult for authorised staff.

This is not the place for a technical dissertation on the security of computer systems, but certain fairly obvious points can be made which will be relevant to most medical systems:*

1. There should be a well-documented data security policy; all employees with access to the system should be aware of their responsibilities.
2. There should be a list of authorised users, each of whom should be the subject of preliminary screening and on-going audit.
3. Equipment (central units and terminals; disks and tapes) should be kept in areas which are either constantly supervised, or which are securely closed if left unattended (e.g. at night). It should be remembered that cables can be 'tapped' – this being very simple for twisted-pairs but almost impossible with fibre-optic links.
4. Access to the computer from a terminal should only be possible after entry of a password. Limited-level access is appropriate in some cases: an appointments clerk does not need to see personal medical data. Associated procedures include automatic disconnection after a number of failed access attempts, and an automatic callback system for use with modems.
5. Transmission of information over multi-user lines should be in a 'scrambled' form. This applies particularly to transmission via modems over the public telephone network.
6. The system should maintain a continuous and comprehensive audit of all user activity.

None of the above will prevent access by an unauthorised but sophisticated user. Equally, however, the situation is no worse than that which obtains with most paper records. Indeed, since people tend to make specific provision for the security of electronic systems, they are usually superior to manuscript notes in this respect.

Data access

A separate but related issue is whether individuals have the right to have access to personal data about themselves held in computer systems. It

---

* *Guidelines on Good Security Practice* is available from BISL Publications, 7-3/4 Delta Business Park, Welton Road, Swindon SN5 7XS, UK.

Table 4.7. Information required from users of clinical data collection systems in the UK according to the Data Protection Act 1984

The name and address of the data user.

A description of the personal data to be held and the purposes for which such data will be used.

A description of the source from which those data will be collected.

A description of any person to whom the data may be disclosed by the user.

Any countries to which those data may be sent.

An address which those persons wishing to see those data may approach.

---

now seems to be almost universally agreed that individuals do have this right, with rare exceptions for certain criminal or political factors where the rights of society as a whole must take precedence. The right of access certainly extends to the individual's own medical records, and there is little reason why this should not be the case, despite some countervailing views from within the profession. These rights are now encapsulated in the law of many nations including the Freedom of Information Acts in the US and the Data Protection Act in the UK (Hayes 1985).*

The practical implications of these rules go beyond a simple awareness that patients can elect to see their own records. In Europe it is also mandated that all electronic systems in which data are held must be registered with a central authority (Table 4.7); failure to comply with such registration requirements is the subject of quite stringent penalties. Furthermore, the authority is responsible for ensuring that all such systems meet certain minimum standards, comparable to those already listed above. In the US there is a wide variation in practice between different states (see White 1986).

Clinical research information systems

Data collected for use in the clinical management of an individual patient can also be used for research purposes: to assemble observations or sets of observations from large numbers of patients. However, it is frequently found that a perfectly satisfactory prospective system (i.e. geared to collection of data for individual patient management) proves to be poorly structured for subsequent retrospective statistical analysis. These problems may be partly avoided, or at least anticipated, if data collection and

---

* In the UK, full information on the requirements of the Act, together with application forms for registration under the Act, can be obtained from any Post Office, or from the Data Protection Registrar, Springfield House, Water Lane, Wilmslow, Cheshire SK9 5AX, UK.

Table 4.8. Examples of statistical software packages which are widely used for medical applications. The criteria for choice of a system have been reviewed in detail by Chan & Portnoy (1988)

Package	Supplier
BMDP	BMDP Statistical Software Inc 1440 Sepulveda Boulevard Los Angeles, CA 90025, USA.
SPSS (Statistical Package for Social Sciences)	SPSS UK Ltd 9–11 Queens Road Walton-on-Thames KT12 5LU, UK.
Statgraphics	Cocking & Drury (Software) Ltd 16 Berkeley Street London W1X 5AE, UK.
SYSTAT	Systat Inc 2902 Central Street Evanston, Illinois 60201, USA.
Minitab	Minitab Inc 3081 Enterprise Drive State College PA 16801, USA.
SAS	SAS Software Ltd Wittington House Henley Road Medmenham Marlow SL7 2EB UK.

data analysis are considered simultaneously during the initial design phase of a system.

Data models

A data model is a description of the relationships among data items. Data models are now widely advocated for use in health care management and clinical data collection. In the UK a very extensive data model covering some 200 separate functions has been developed; this is known as the Common Basic Specification (CBS) (Molteno & Bishop 1988).

Statistical packages

Information collected from a database can be analysed using a number of widely available statistical packages. All the packages listed in Table 4.8 have a facility for entry of data in tabular form: either via its own editor, or by importing ASCII files from word processors, databases or spreadsheets. All provide a full range of descriptive and analytical statistics. They differ somewhat in ease of use and sophistication of graphic output.

Table 4.9. Examples of specialised clinical data collection systems

Application	Reference
Psychological assessment	Fowler 1985
Sexual assessment	Barnard et al. 1987
Health risk appraisal	Black & Ashton 1985
Assessment of reading difficulties and language deficits	Ray 1985
Assessment of dietary intake	Levine et al. 1987
Fertility/Infertility	Lilford et al. 1983 Duisterhout & Schoemaker 1987
Perinatal medicine	Chard 1990a Yoong et al. 1993
Memory tests	Corwin & Snodgrass 1987
Triage in the emergency department	Berman et al. 1989
Back pain	Thomas et al. 1989

Specialised data collection systems

There are certain repetitive and well-structured data collection functions which lend themselves particularly well to automation (Table 4.9). Prominent among these is psychological assessment and the application of computers to this function is often referred to as 'computer-based test interpretation' or CBTI. These systems were among the first medical data applications for computers, having been used as part of psychometric testing since the 1950s (see Fowler 1985)*. The best known of these systems is the Minnesota Multiphasic Personality Inventory (MMPI)†, intelligence tests, social history, and depression inventories are also often included. The MMPI was originally computerised at the Mayo Clinic and was based on special cards that were marked by the patient and then optically scanned for entry into a mainframe computer. Subsequent developments (as in other areas of computing) including an increasing use of on-line, interactive questioning, and the production of narrative reports derived from the test scores. As in other areas of computer data collection, patient reaction to CBTI is generally favourable (French & Beaumont 1987).

---

* A series of articles on this topic appeared in the *Journal of Consulting and Clinical Psychology* (Vol. 53, No. 6, 1985).
† Currently available from NCS Professional Assessment Services, PO Box 1416, Dept 375, Minneapolis, MN 55440, USA.

5

Computers and medical diagnosis

A computer system can make diagnoses as well as (but not better than) most humans. The great potential strength of the machine is that its performance is the same at all times and on all sites. The weakness is that few practical systems are currently available, and that these apply only to relatively narrow clinical fields. This is an area in which new technology ('artificial intelligence') has been much overpraised.

The major applications of computers in medicine are the collection, storage and retrieval of information. However, the very nature of the machine opens the possibility of its use to draw conclusions from complex data. In medicine, these conclusions are the 'diagnosis' and this, in turn, defines the action which is 'treatment'.

As soon as a computer system goes beyond being a simple passive receptacle for information it acquires characteristics which, because they mimic some aspects of human thought, have variously been described as 'expert systems' or 'artificial intelligence'.

Expert systems

Expert systems can be defined as the 'embodiment within a computer of knowledge from an expert skill in such a form that the system can offer intelligent advice or take an intelligent decision'. Some would argue that the definition of an expert system should also include the capability of self-explanation. However, this makes the definition too stringent and would exclude virtually every medical process which has so far been described as an expert system.

Artificial intelligence

Artificial intelligence (AI) has been defined as 'behaviour by a machine which would be regarded as intelligent if it were performed by a human'. The characteristics of an AI system may also include the abilities of self-learning and for explaining the reasoning underlying a given conclusion. Another attractive definition is that it is an expert system which is capable of developing itself.

The definition of artificial intelligence is often broadened to include functions such as vision and language recognition. However, these are best placed in a separate category of 'artificial perception'. Thus, they are perfectly well developed in species (e.g. dogs) which would not typically be accepted as intelligent in the sense that they should be emulated in a medical diagnostic system.

Artificial perception

Perceptive functions (notably hearing and vision) are universal among humans, almost regardless of the level of intelligence, but have proved formidably difficult to emulate with a computer. It can be safely predicted that for the foreseeable future (i.e. in this century) there will be no routine, practical system of two-way verbal exchange between patient and machine. Similarly, though the machine analysis of complex digitised images has great potential in investigative medicine, this does not extend to the sort of pattern recognition which will immediately tell any other human that the patient is in pain.

Application of expert systems to the clinical process

Expert systems can be applied to any part of the clinical process – data collection, diagnosis, or treatment (Fig. 5.1). Thus, in a data collection system, the expertise (knowledge) lies in knowing which questions to ask and in what order. The sequence of questions (decisions) may be entirely predetermined or, more often, may be determined by a series of branches based on the response to individual questions. However, the term 'expert system' is most commonly used to describe the process whereby conclusions are reached from data which have already been collected. It is this meaning which is adopted here.

Clinical diagnosis by computer

What is a diagnosis?

A diagnosis is a word or set of words which describes a group of clinical features; the latter may be symptoms, signs, results of special investigations and pathological examination, or some combination of these. A diagnosis is, in effect, a brief summary of a case which identifies it with other cases having a similar underlying pathology and distinguishes it from those which do not. In operational terms it serves as a convenient label on the basis of which all subsequent management will be predicted. Reaching a diagnosis is at the ultimate core of all professional medical practice.

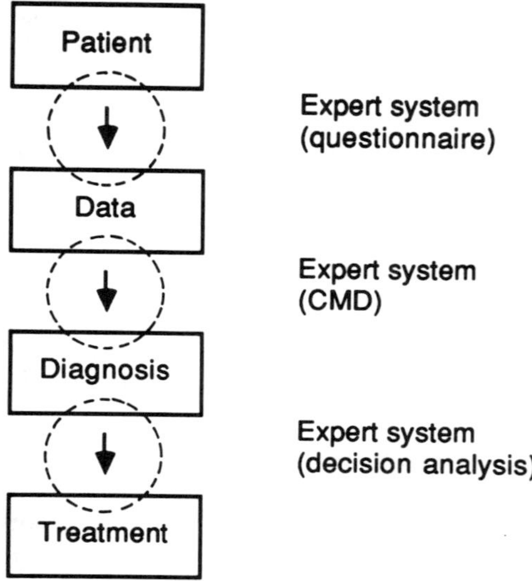

Fig. 5.1.   The applications of expert systems to the clinical process. Any of the main steps may be the subject of an expert system, but the term is usually reserved for the use of the computer in diagnosis and treatment.

Some diagnoses may be of extreme simplicity, where a single presenting feature may also be the final conclusion.* For example, a patient who states 'I have an in-growing toenail' may well have just that condition: the presenting feature and the diagnosis are identical and the only contribution which could be made by a machine would be to record the facts of the situation. Much more commonly, however, a diagnosis represents the conclusion reached from a multiplicity of features. Furthermore, much of the information collected in the earlier stages of evaluation of a case will be non-definitive: for example, the complaint of a 'painful swollen toe' and even the observation of a painful swollen toe might be compatible with a diagnosis of an in-growing toenail, but are also compatible with a number of alternative diagnoses (gout, foreign body, etc.). Virtually all of medical diagnosis consists of a process of reaching a conclusion of more or less certainty from a multiplicity of clinical features none of which, on its own, is definitive.

---

* Blois (1984) has suggested that the attributes of a disease can be described at one or more of ten hierarchical levels, where the whole body is the highest level and atoms are the lowest levels. The highest levels are the area of the patient's complaint (e.g. anorexia, malaise) while the physician tries to focus the diagnosis to the lowest possible level (tissue, cell or molecule). Higher level attributes tend to be fuzzy, sharpness increases at lower levels.

'Absolute' diagnosis versus operational diagnosis

In a perfect world the aim of clinical medicine would be to achieve the best possible diagnosis in every case. 'Best', in this sense, would mean the diagnosis with the highest degree of likelihood having excluded all other possibilities. Reality dictates that most diagnoses fall short of this optimum. The patient reporting to a general practitioner with a one-day old headache will be asked a few simple questions and prescribed analgesia: the elaborate investigations necessary to prove or exclude a cerebral tumour are highly unlikely at this stage. The operational diagnosis is 'headache', implicit in which is the qualifying adjective 'simple' or 'benign'.

The importance of distinguishing between operational and absolute diagnoses is that in real-life clinical practice most diagnoses are operational. However, designers of computer-diagnosis systems (often a committee of designers) are always tempted towards the absolute, and consequently end up with procedures which are theoretically sound but impractical. Computer experts are often unaware that a given diagnosis may exist at a variety of different levels, and that an important medical skill is knowing not just what facts to obtain, but also when to stop acquiring information.

It is also important to recognise that most clinical information is non-definitive, i.e. the findings may be associated with a number of different diagnoses. Much less common are findings which are pathognomonic (providing absolute confirmation of diagnosis), or exclusionary (absolutely ruling out a diagnosis), or obligatory (absence of the finding rules out the diagnosis).

Analytical versus synthetic reasoning in medical diagnosis

An important aspect of the emulation of human performance by a computer is the route by which a conclusion is reached. There are two approaches which in formal logic are usually defined as 'analytical' and 'synthetic' (see also Elstein et al. 1978). In the analytical approach a series of facts are collected which are then assembled to draw a conclusion. In the synthetic or hypothetico-deductive approach the first step is the conclusion, after which facts are sought which might confirm or refute that conclusion. In the purely analytical approach a patient with a headache would be asked all relevant questions and subjected to all relevant examinations, before a diagnosis was made. The synthetic approach is well illustrated by the real-life physician faced with a patient with headache: he may immediately have a 'hunch' that this is a case of brain tumour, and will then confine his initial questioning and investigation to that possibility.* Human diagnosis is usually some combination of analytical and synthetic although, very correctly, it is the analytical approach which is taught in medical schools while the synthetic approach is left to develop with experience.

The relevant point about this distinction is that computer diagnosis is almost inevitably weighted towards the analytical approach – the meticulous accumulation of facts in the absence of preconceived ideas. The great strength of the machine is its ability to follow complex but predetermined paths of data collection, and then to draw mathematically accurate conclusions. However, some designers of computer diagnosis systems do attempt to emulate the synthetic, intuitive human approach. They then rapidly discover that they need immensely sophisticated equipment capable (like the human brain) of parallel operation: at the present time such equipment, where it is available at all, is impractically expensive. The dangers of slavish emulation by a computer have been nicely illustra⁺ed by the analogy of flight: a real life bird may be better designed than a fixed-wing aircraft, but the latter provides an immensely successful means of transport.

Methods for computer-assisted medical decision making

There are many different approaches to computer-assisted medical decision making (CMD). These have been reviewed in detail by Reggia & Tuhrim (1985) and the discussion here follows the lines set out by these authors. The fundamental components of a CMD system are shown in Fig. 5.2. This structure has also been used to classify the humans associated with a CMD system. Those physicians who provide the knowledge base are the 'medical experts' or 'knowledge base authors'; the computer scientists who design the inference engine are 'knowledge engineers'; and the physicians who will apply the system are the 'users'. The methods applied have also been divided into a number of groups (Table 5.1) and these are reviewed in turn here.

Algorithmic methods

An algorithm is a series of step-by-step instructions on how to perform some task. Probably the majority of successful current CMD systems are based on this approach (see Table 5.6). The obvious advantages are that it is conceptually very simple, and that it is very easily implemented using standard procedural languages (FORTRAN, BASIC, Pascal). In BASIC, for example, the instructions are a series of statements on successive lines,

---

* Human memory restricts consideration of hypotheses to four ± one at any one time (Elstein et al. 1972)

Table 5.1. A classification of methods used in CMD systems (from Reggia & Tuhrim 1985)

Algorithmic methods
Statistical pattern classification
Production rule systems
Cognitive models

---

with conditional branches to other lines where appropriate. Conclusions (diagnosis or therapy) are reached by one or more 'if ... then' statements: 'if' the patient has clinical features X and Y, but not Z, 'then' the diagnosis is probably condition A and the treatment is drug 1 (Fig. 5.3). With algorithmic systems of this type the inference engine is, in effect, the program language.

Although the algorithmic systems might appear simple and attractive they are not especially popular in the community of researchers in CMD. Disadvantages are said to include the lack of precise quantitative formulas for many medical problems, and the absence of a clear distinction between the knowledge base and the inference engine. However, it is likely that the general popularity and success of algorithmic systems will continue until a system of equal practicality and superior abilities becomes available.

Statistical pattern classification

The best-known procedures under this heading are Bayes' theorem, linear discriminant functions and database comparisons.

Bayes' theorem

The theoretical basis of this very well-known approach to CMD systems was described by a clergyman, Thomas Bayes, in the eighteenth century. In effect, Bayes' theorem, presents all knowledge as a set of probabilities – which explains the theorem's great value in clinical medicine, in which virtually all probabilities are less than 1 (i.e. there is hardly ever total certainty). Bayes' theorem combines the prior probabilities of outcomes together with the conditional probabilities of various input features in order to reach a posterior probability or conclusion. In practical terms, Bayes' theorem can be used to calculate the probability of various diagnoses given the clinical features of an individual patient. This process of drawing conclusions of more or less certainty from multiple pieces of information, none of which is definitive on its own, is an almost perfect description of much of clinical medicine and is the machine equivalent of what is often described as human intuition.

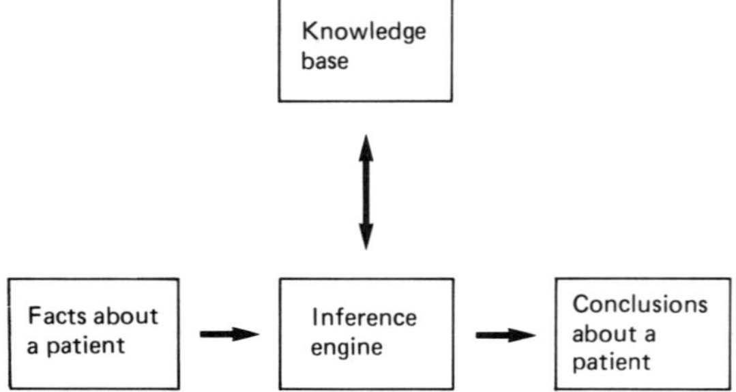

Fig. 5.2.   A diagram of a computer-assisted medical decision-making CMD system (modified from Reggia & Tuhrim 1985). The input is a description of the clinical features of a specific patient; the output is some sort of conclusion which may be a diagnosis and/or suggestions for additional tests and treatment. The knowledge base is a collection of predetermined 'facts' needed to solve problems in a given subject. The inference engine is a program which assembles the information about the patient together with that in the knowledge base and draws a conclusion about the patient.

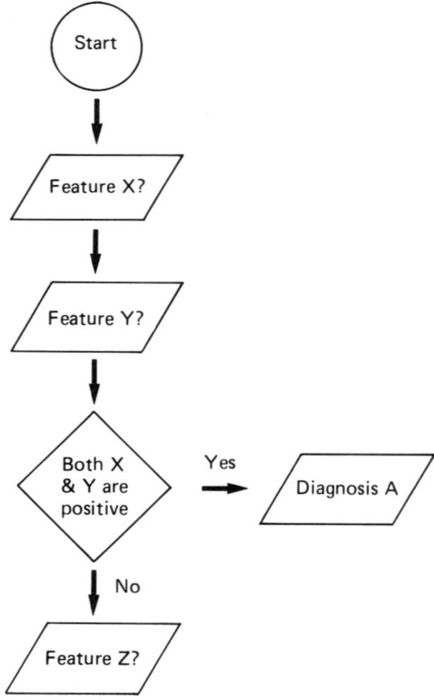

Fig. 5.3.   A diagram to illustrate the algorithmic approach to a CMD. Information is obtained on two clinical features, X and Y. If both are present (positive) then the conclusion of diagnosis A can be reached. If either or both features are negative the program requests another input (feature Z). In real-life, flow-charts of this type are usually of much greater size and complexity. Nevertheless, they are easy to implement using standard languages and equipment.

The equation of Bayes' theorem appears in various forms, one of which is as follows:

$$P(D{:}CF) = \frac{P(CF{:}D)P(D)}{P(CF{:}D)P(D) + P(CF{:}\text{ not }D)P(\text{not }D)} \qquad (5.1)$$

where P is probability, D is diagnosis, and CF is a set of clinical features. Thus the expression on the left, P(D:CF), is equivalent, in words, to 'the probability P of diagnosis D given the set of features CF'. On the right P(D) and P(not D) represent the prior probabilities of the diagnosis and its alternatives.

In a clinical situation there would be a number of possible diagnoses and a number of clinical features. A probability calculation is made for each condition; the 'diagnosis' is the condition with the highest probability. This equation is the 'inference engine' (see Fig. 5.1) of a Bayesian CMD system. The knowledge-base for a given clinical situation consists of a matrix of all the possible diseases and all the clinical findings in these diseases. Each cell in the matrix contains the incidence of the finding in the given disease (P(CF:D)).

Table 5.2. The incidence of clinical features, a and b, in two diseases, X and Y. The two diseases have an equal incidence. For the purposes of the example shown in the text it is assumed that X and Y are mutually exclusive and that a and b are independent

Disease	Incidence of feature (%)	
	a	b
X	10	90
Y	90	10

As the concept of Bayes' theorem is important but not easy for a non-mathematician to grasp at a brief glance, it can be illustrated by a simple worked example. Table 5.2 shows the incidence of two clinical features, a and b, in two diseases, X and Y, which have an equal incidence (i.e. the prior probability, P(D), of each is 0.5). To begin with, take a case in which both features, a and b, are positive, and work out the posterior probability (P(D:CF), of each diagnosis. For diagnosis X this would appear as follows:

$$P(X{:}CF) = \frac{P(a{:}X)P(b{:}X)P(X)}{[P(a{:}X)P(b{:}X)P(X) + (P(A{:}Y)P(b{:}Y)P(Y)]} \qquad (5.2)$$

Note that the expression on the right-hand side of the bottom line, giving the probabilities in respect of diagnosis Y, is in this case the equivalent of 'not D' in equation 5.1. Substitution of the actual numbers in equation 5.2 gives:

$$P(X\!:\!CF) = \frac{0.1 \times 0.9 \times 0.5}{(0.1 \times 0.9 \times 0.5) + (0.9 \times 0.1 \times 0.5)} \qquad (5.3)$$
$$= 0.5$$

Obviously the same conclusion would be reached in respect of P(Y:CF). The answer to this particular example might be considered so obvious as not to require recondite mathematics. That would be true for this case, but not for situations in which there are multiple possible diagnoses with different frequencies and multiple clinical features; as the complexity increases, so the answer becomes less obvious and the mathematical approach correspondingly becomes more valuable.

For the final example take a case in which a is positive but b is not. Then:

$$P(X\!:\!CF) = \frac{P(a\!:\!X)P(not\ b\!:\!X)P(X)}{[(P(a\!:\!X)P(not\ b\!:\!X)P(X)] + [(P(a\!:\!Y)P(not\ b\!:\!Y)P(Y)]} \qquad (5.3)$$
$$= 0.012$$

This answer, though factually correct, is rather less obvious than that of the previous example.

Some practical aspects of the use of Bayes' theorem

There are certain rules on the use of Bayes' theorem of which potential users should be aware:

1. Bayes' theorem can never give an absolute and definitive diagnosis (or if it does, it is being used incorrectly). It merely assigns a probability to each of the possible diagnoses and, typically, the conclusion with the highest probability is 'the diagnosis'.
2. The possible diagnoses must be mutually exclusive. For example 'headache' and 'brain tumour' in the same list would not be acceptable, whereas 'brain tumour' and 'temporal arteritis' would be acceptable. An obvious problem is that an individual patient may have multiple diagnoses; Bayes' theorem cannot assist with this, other than by the fact that it never excludes a diagnosis.
3. The clinical features should be independent of each other. For example, the urinary symptoms of 'urgency' and 'frequency' are so closely linked that it is probably incorrect to incorporate them as separate items. In reality, however, it can be difficult to establish that given features are truly independent and even more so to quantitate

this factor. Fortunately, the outcome of Bayesian calculations is not drastically affected by some measure of dependence and within reasonable limits this rule can be ignored (see Chard 1989).

4. The clinical features must be binary, i.e. present or absent. It is usually not too difficult to achieve this, even for numerical information, simply by specifying a cut-off point, for example, 'diastolic blood pressure above 90 mmHg – yes or no'. Similarly the outcomes may be a single diagnosis with some appropriate subclassification, for example, 'good'. 'fair' or 'poor' recovery from a stroke or heart attack.

5. As with all CMD systems, the efficiency of Bayes' theorem is very dependent on the accuracy of the knowledge base.

6. It is often found that Bayes' theorem gives the best results with a subset of the total diagnostic information (Chard and Rubenstein 1989). For example, in a study on a CMD system for jaundice it was found that only 22 of a total of 107 variables originally collected were necessary to achieve optimum results (Malchow-Moller et al. 1986). Indeed, consideration of an excessive number of variables may actually decrease the efficiency of the procedure.

Linear discriminant functions

In this approach various clinical features are given a numerical value. The data are then used to create a linear equation (i.e. the numbers are added together). The result is a 'discriminant function' which serves to divide the relevant population into two or more parts. Various different forms of discriminant analysis have been described and the topic can be highly confusing to the non-mathematician. Fortunately, the choice of approach seems to make little difference to the eventual clinical results (Titterington et al. 1981). Overall, discriminant analysis has the same features as those already described for Bayes' theorem.

Database comparisons

In this method a new patient is compared with previous similar patients in a clinical database (Feinstein et al. 1972; Haberman et al. 1985). The principle of this is illustrated in Fig. 5.4. This is the approach used in so-called bitmap systems (e.g. QMR). Each diagnosis is stored as a bitmap (array of 0s and 1s). Thus two diseases might be reported as 1010000 and 1010111. Faced with a new case, the expert system uses pattern matching to find the closest fit. The latter is taken into account by estimating a 'distance' between the patient and the database. The inability to identify an exact relationship between an individual patient and a knowledge base is also dealt with in the branch of mathematics known as 'fuzzy set theory' (Zadeh 1968).

DATABASE COMPARISON

	a	b	c	d
X	+	+	+	+
Y	+	+	−	+
Z	−	+	+	+

Fig. 5.4. Diagram to illustrate the principle of clinical diagnosis by database comparison. Four clinical features (a to d) define the presence or absence of three diagnoses (X, Y and Z). A patient positive for all four features would therefore have diagnosis X. In practice the situation is far more complex because 'presence or absence' is usually a probability rather than a certainty. The database would contain numerous examples of X, Y and Z, and the result would be presented as that diagnosis which most frequently presented the same features as the current case.

The advantage of CMD systems based on database comparisons is that they make no assumption as to the independence or otherwise of the clinical features. Disadvantages include the requirement for a very large database, especially if it is to contain representative examples of rare conditions, and that the system is not workable until the database has been accumulated at considerable effort and expense. Furthermore, the depth and extent of the database search places heavy demands on the computer hardware. The major argument in favour of large databases is that they provide hard information, as opposed to opinions, on the frequency estimates used for Bayes' theorem.

Production rule systems

Production rule systems are the first of the CMD systems which come under the heading of what professionals would regard as artificial intelligence. In production rule systems each rule/production has the form 'IF antecedents THEN consequents': if the antecedent conditions are true then the consequents are also true (see Fig. 5.5). The inference engine of this type of system is an interpreter which examines sets of rules in the knowledge base in relation to the features of a particular case.

How does this differ from a simple algorithmic system, since at first glance the two might appear remarkably similar, not to say identical? The answer resides in the terms 'procedural' and 'non-procedural'. An algorithmic system is procedural and follows predetermined paths. In the example shown in Fig. 5.5 an algorithmic system would call for an input of 'age?': the next step would be conditional branch 'IF age = 35 or 36 then recommendation' or 'IF age 35 or 36 then next step'. A production rule system, by contrast, is non-procedural. Following an input of age (say 36) the knowledge base is searched in its entirety to ascertain whether there are any rules triggered by this information. If there are, the

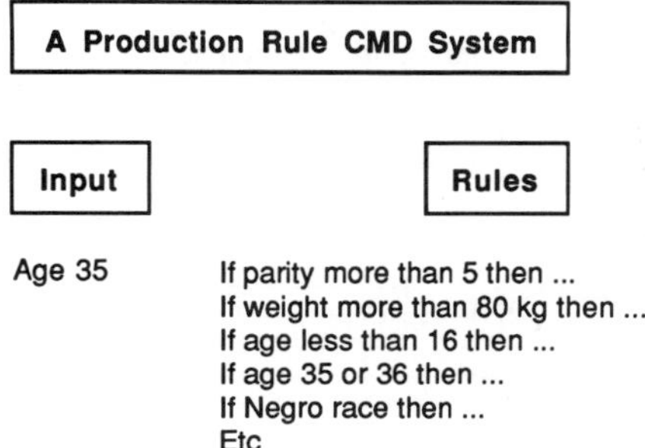

Fig. 5.5. An example of a production rule from a CMD system providing advice on screening tests in pregnancy. Note that rules of this type are not branching points in a program but are simple statements of fact.

consequents are displayed; if there are not, the program moves to the next step.

The difference between algorithmic and production rule systems is illustrated in Figs 5.6 and 5.7. So far as the user is concerned, entry of age will trigger the same recommendation from both systems. However, entry of 'red hair' would bring an algorithmic system to a halt because there would be no procedural step of the 'IF red hair then ...' type. By contrast, a production rule system would search its knowledge base, discover that there were no rules concerning red hair, if necessary announce that fact, and then pass on to the next step.

The advantage of a production rule CMD system is that rules of the sort shown in Fig. 5.5 can be added more or less ad infinitum without needing to be related to specific inputs: the program will find them anyway. The most obvious disadvantage is that, in a practical system, large numbers of rules will have to be searched following each and every entry. Large numbers of rules are needed in order to allow for the context of the

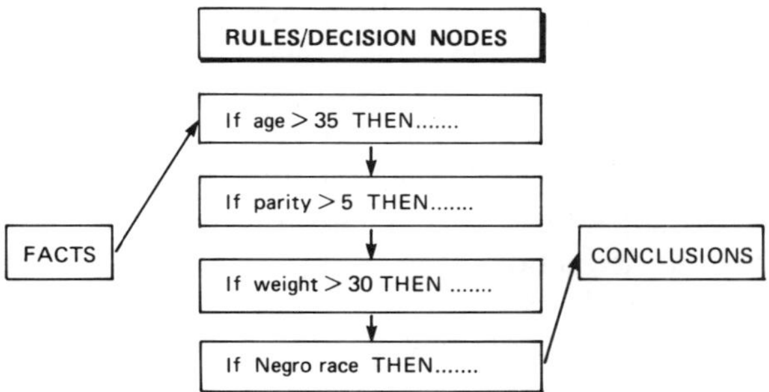

Fig. 5.6. Algorithmic system. If the system is at a decision node that requires the input 'age', it can continue only after the 'age' has been provided. If other information is given the system will come to a halt because there is a predetermined sequence which *must* be followed. (Modified from Chard & Schreiner 1990.)

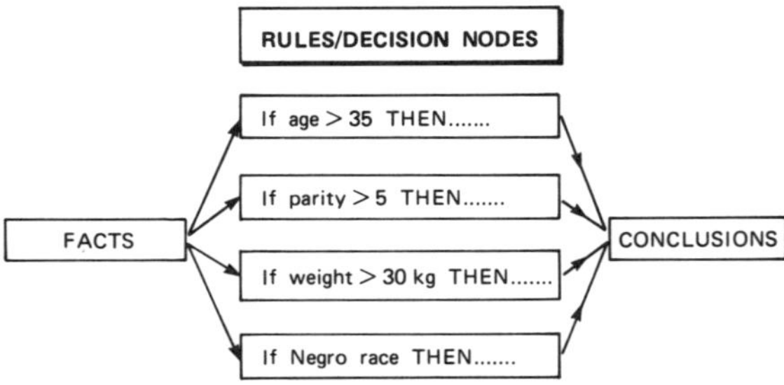

Fig. 5.7.   Production rule system. Of all the possible routes through the system, the inference engine chooses the one most appropriate to a given input. If no relevant input is available, the system will simply continue with the next step. (Modified from Chard & Schreiner 1990.)

information, for example, the rule in Fig. 5.5 would not be true if the patient were seeking termination of pregnancy on social grounds, or was more than 20 weeks pregnant. In real life it is usually far easier and quicker for the human expert to determine the context, or that 'red hair' is not relevant and therefore exclude it from valid inputs, than to go on a long complex search which may prove fruitless. Another disadvantage is that medical knowledge tends to be organised in a descriptive manner, and reformulation into a complete set of discrete rules can be a formidable task.

There are a number of variants on production rule CMD systems:

1. Forward-chaining versus backward-chaining: The systems described above are forward-chaining (also referred to as antecedent-driven or bottom-up inductive). They begin with features of a case and work forward to conclusions. However, these systems can just as easily work in reverse. They are then described as backward-chaining (consequent-driven, top down, deductive) (Figs 5.8 and 5.9). A conclusion is selected and then the data which might confirm or disprove that conclusion are sought. Forward chaining is most useful with a small set of relevant facts. Backward chaining is most appropriate with a large set of facts, where one fact can yield many conclusions.

2. Rules may be assembled as a 'chain' or decision-tree in order to make multi-step deductions (for example, in a system for leukaemia diagnosis; Alvey et al. 1987a).

3. Rules may be absolute, or may include an element of uncertainty (probability).

4. Rules, once triggered, can easily be made to document themselves, thus providing a 'self-explanatory' function.

Some of the best known of the earlier CMD systems were of the production rule type, for example MYCIN for the choice of antibiotic therapy (Davis et al. 1977), ONCOCIN for cancer therapy, PUFF for the interpretation of pulmonary function tests, and CASNET/GLAUCOMA for diagnosis of glaucoma (Weiss et al. 1978).

A feature of the knowledge-base of some production-rule systems is causal reasoning. The knowledge is represented as a network of diseases and clinical findings, together with the causal relationships among these which may include cause-of, caused-by, develops-into and complication-of. Any disease can be described as a pattern within this network. Furthermore, the causal knowledge is arranged in different hierarchies, for example, one hierarchical level would describe the involvement of individual organs, another would increase the detail to the time level. Causal representation is said to enable a basic understanding of a disease process. However, it is formidably difficult to understand, to construct and to program.

Cognitive models

Cognitive models represent the further reaches of the AI spectrum and are an attempt to model, as closely as possible, the reasoning of human diagnosticians. The commonest approach to the construction of such a model is to record a clinical interview and then to 'debrief' the clinician as to the thought process involved ('thinking aloud'). This always confirms that human diagnostic reasoning consists of a series of hypothesise-and-test steps during the course of which the physician constructs a conceptual model of the patient (Fig. 5.10). Elstein has classified these activities as cue acquisition, hypothesis generation, cue interpretation, and hypothesis calculation.

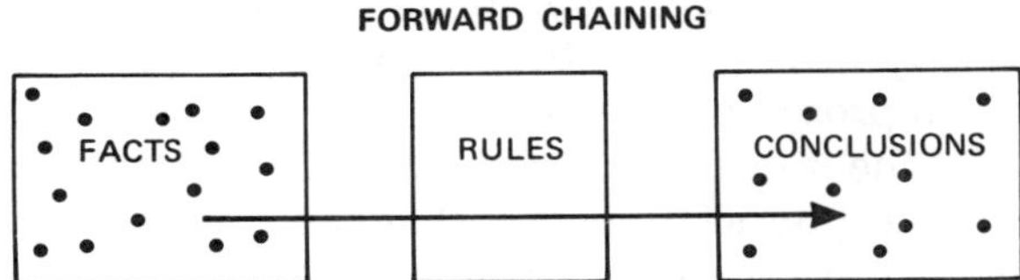

Fig. 5.8. Forward chaining. From the facts available, *all* possible conclusions are searched for and derived. (Modified from Chard & Schreiner 1990.)

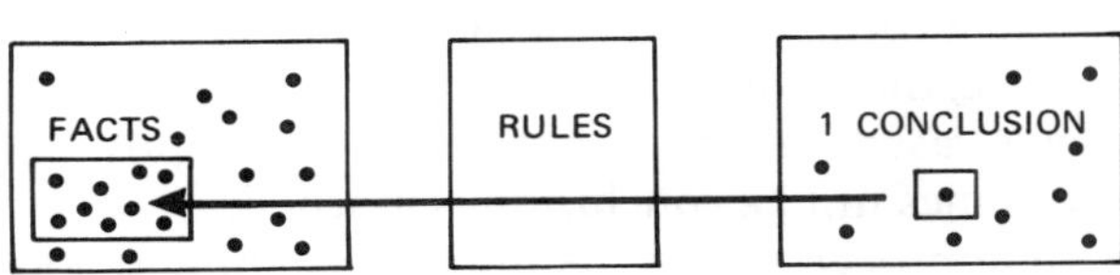

Fig. 5.9. Backward chaining. The system searches only for the data it needs to confirm or disprove the one conclusion under consideration. (Modified from Chard & Schreiner 1990.)

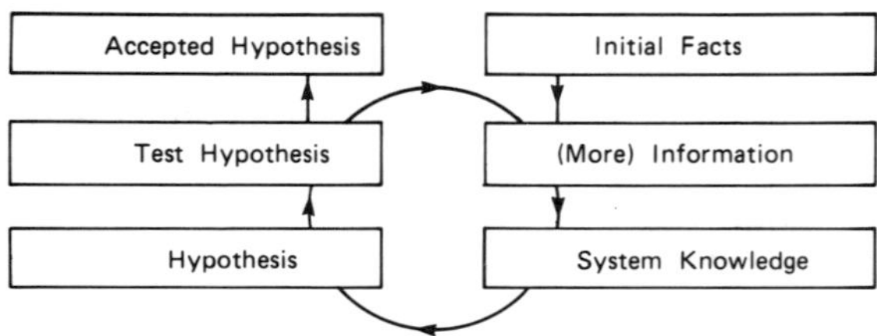

Fig. 5.10. Diagram to illustrate the principle of the cognitive model approach to a CMD system. As the result of input of information the physician forms a hypothesis about a patient (the hypothesis is a sort of intermediate, working diagnosis selected from a number of competing explanations of the patient's problems). Further information is then sought in order to strengthen or repudiate the hypothesis. At some, usually rather indeterminate point, the process is concluded and the final hypothesis becomes the actual diagnosis. It has been estimated that this occurs when the clinician has assembled about 70 per cent of the potentially useful data (Feightner 1975). (Modified from Chard & Schreiner 1990.)

At an early stage of the process there are usually multiple hypotheses (differential diagnosis). The natural human aim is to reduce the number of diagnoses to the minimum, often one, which will satisfactorily explain the patient's problems; this goal of the minimum is sometimes referred to as Occam's razor.

At all stages in the process the physician will attempt to rank a piece of information or a hypothesis according to its usefulness or likelihood. It is an interesting fact that the human mind tends to use only a three-point system for ranking – in effect, 'yes', 'no' or 'perhaps' (Elstein et al. 1978). So a diagnosis may be highly probable (say 0.95 to 1.0 on a probability scale), or highly improbable (say 0.00 to 0.05), or somewhere in-between; the probability of the in-between category could be anywhere from 0.05 to 0.95 without the physician feeling that there was any very strong weighting one way or the other. Fortunately, a 3-point scale can often yield the same diagnostic efficiency as absolute probability (Chard 1991).

The knowledge base of a cognitive model consists of 'frames' of associated information; such frames are thought to be a reflection of the organisation of memory in the human. For example, a frame might consist of the name of a test, the principle conditions in which it is positive or negative, the hazards and the costs. The inference engine of a cognitive model is based on a hypothesise-and-test approach, i.e. cycling through sets of frames until a conclusion is reached.

A well-known approach which fits into the cognitive model group is the so-called problem knowledge coupler (Weed & Hertzberg 1984; Pollock 1986). In this the clinician seeks a principal finding or problem ('pivotal sign') and then considers all the causes of that problem, ranking them according to how well they account for other patient findings and attributes. This somewhat idiosyncratic approach is apparently successful in veterinary practice, where there is often a single and obvious presenting feature (e.g. coughing, itching, vomiting).

The major problem of cognitive models is that they can become extraordinarily complex if they are to take account of the apparent human ability to deal with multiple simultaneous hypotheses. It is this type of parallel reasoning which has led some to conclude that similar structures will be needed in medical computer hardware, at a cost proportional to the nth power of the number of simultaneous processes. Another problem is the very obvious differences in thought processes likely to be encountered among human experts of equivalent ability. It would seem slightly ridiculous to build this variability into a CMD system.

Neural networks

An area of AI research which has received much publicity is the use of neural networks or neurocomputers (Reggia 1988; Stubbs 1988). These are systems composed of a network of neuron-like processing devices. Computations are performed in parallel by each element, so that collectively the network provides enormous computational power. Extensive feedback ensures that the system is capable of learning. The system achieves this by altering the strength of the connections between processors according to the results obtained. Furthermore, the network serves both as memory and processor, unlike conventional AI systems (Fig. 5.2) in which these functions are distinct.

Neural networks can run on PCs, but run much faster on devices such as the Connection Machine which has many thousands of simple processors, each with its own memory, embedded in a communication network. Software is rather more problematic: most programs for biomedical work are at the research rather than the application state. Pattern recognition for imaging and signal processing are thought to be important potential uses (Dytch & Wied 1990). One research area of great interest is the use of these machines to model neurophysiological events in the brain, especially the architecture of the visual cortex (Linsker 1986). However, construction of a machine equivalent to the whole human brain is likely to prove more difficult since the brain is a network of 5×10^{10} neurons (processors) with 1014 synapses (communication channels).*

---

* A housefly would be simpler with only 10^6 neurons, or better still a worm with 10^3 neurons.

The present place of artificial intelligence

Artificial intelligence has had a bad press in the recent past. This is at least partly justified by earlier over-confidence in the topic. However, so far as clinical medicine is concerned, there is little doubt that the concepts of AI can make a major practical contribution (Szolovits et al. 1988). There is also no doubt that for the foreseeable future AI will in no sense replace the human professional (Schwartz et al. 1986).

Table 5.3. Examples of jargon which have been used to describe various concepts of artificial intelligence. The unnecessary use of some of these obscure terms has brought the subject a measure of disrepute

Heuristic	A 'rule of thumb'. A rule which is probable rather than definitive, but in which the probability is poorly defined.
Community	A group or people using a common set of jargon.
Graceful degradation	The computer, faced with a problem it cannot solve, presents a polite and understandable message and suggestions for alternative approaches.
Deep, rich	A simple system multiplied to such an extent that it becomes incomprehensible.

One of the major criticisms of AI is that its concepts have been wrapped in obscure terminology largely, some feel, to exclude the subject from consideration by all but a small group of practitioners. This is a perfectly fair objection: some examples of the jargon which has been employed are shown in Table 5.3. Other problems include:

1. Views on AI are often coloured by experience with earlier systems: MYCIN and others were brilliant prototypes but for practical purposes are now of historic interest only.

2. The transition from a prototype demonstrator system to a practical high-performance system can present many problems. A small system which works well cannot simply be scaled up without introducing gross errors in complex and difficult cases. This was well-illustrated in an EMYCIN system for leukaemia diagnosis (Alvey et al. 1987b).

Defining the knowledge base for CMD systems

A major problem in setting up a CMD system is to define and produce the knowledge base. For the statistical systems knowledge must be numerically accurate or at least approximate to such accuracy (Chard 1991). For the non-procedural, AI type of approach numerical accuracy is less essential, but it has to be recognised that the conclusions cannot be more accurate than the knowledge base. For example, if the knowledge base contains the item 'X is probably the result of Y' then 'probably Y' is also the best conclusion that the machine can reach. It cannot, as if by magic, turn this into 'there is a 60 per cent chance that X is the result of Y'.

A perfect knowledge base would contain all the known and possible features of a clinical situation, together with the quantitative relationships amongst those features.* For example, in the case of a 50-year-old with persistent headaches the knowledge base would contain a list of possible diagnoses and the frequency of each, together with the frequency of each clinical feature in each diagnosis. Unfortunately, complete information of this type is only rarely available in any field of clinical medicine. Indeed, for most situations (such as the headache example above) not more than 30 or 40 per cent of the information would be available in usable numerical form.

There are four main approaches to the development of a knowledge base:

1. *Use of an existing database.* Typically, this would be information derived from published data in a journal or textbook. The disadvantage of this approach is that the information is often incomplete, particularly in respect of the frequency of various clinical features; furthermore, the information may not apply to the local population for which the system is intended.

2. *Development of a new database based on local practice.* The so-called case-based systems can be very efficient. If complete information is available on the previous one thousand 50-year-olds with headache, the machine can derive executable rules from these examples and apply them to the features in the current subject. Unfortunately, the construction of such a database consumes large amounts of time and resources prior to yielding a useful product. This is a situation which may improve with the increasing trend towards electronic collection of clinical data.

3. *Development of a database as part of the actual use of an expert system.* In other words the machine develops its own knowledge base from data which it acquires as part of its operation in routine clinical practice – a process described as 'bootstrapping'. The problem with this approach is that the knowledge base will not become effective until substantial numbers of cases have accumulated, and it may be difficult to judge when this point has been reached (Chard 1987a).

---

* Knowledge is sometimes divided into declarative and procedural. Declarative knowledge describes objects and events; procedural knowledge describes actions and relationships.

4. *The 'Delphic' system*. This is the approach in which the necessary knowledge is generated by seeking the opinions of 'experts'. It is fairly rapid and simple, but often re-confirms the well-known fact that experts differ widely in their opinion of numerical information which superficially would appear to be straightforward and familiar (Dolan et al. 1986). Furthermore, physicians are often unfamiliar with the concept of probability estimates. Most humans can only conceive probability as a 3-point scale: probably (0.9–1.0); possible (0.1–0.9); and unlikely (0–0.1). However, even semi-quantitative estimates can be helpful (Chard 1991). Attempts to evaluate the probabilistic judgement of physicians is now a research area in its own right (Poses et al. 1988) and a program had been described to train physicians in probability estimation (Fryback 1986). Interestingly, experts tend to produce knowledge-bases which are smaller and less complex than those of non-experts (Leao & Roche 1990). The problem of disagreement amongst experts can sometimes be solved by repeated rounds of consultation (Kors et al. 1990).

In real-life, development of the knowledge base for a CMD system is usually a mixture of all these approaches. The knowledge engineer, faced with the patient with headache, would first examine textbooks and list all possible diagnoses and the clinical features associated with each of these diagnoses. He would also ascertain those numerical facts which are readily available in the literature. He would assemble all this information in a table which would, of course, have numerous gaps. At this point he would sit down with a human expert – a specialist neurologist – and ask that expert to give estimates for all the missing information. If the expert cannot be persuaded to give a single figure (e.g. 40 per cent) then he should be asked to suggest a range (e.g. 30 to 50 per cent). Whatever range is suggested, the median is taken as the actual value. Finally, the validity of the whole process is much enhanced if a number of experts can be examined so that the end-result is a consensus rather than an individual view (Schreiner & Chard 1991).

The knowledge-base as a diagnostic support system

The knowledge-base of an expert system can be of great value as a diagnostic aide-memoire without itself drawing any conclusions. Examples of this include QUICK (QUick Index to Caduceus Knowledge; First et al. 1985; Miller et al. 1992) and ASK*MED (Bernstein et al. 1980). ASK*MED consists of an extensive and detailed clinical text. On the basis of a query this text is searched for all associated items and paragraphs, ranked according to their relevance to the query. Systems of this type do not aim to provide a model of clinical judgement but rather to provide a compact, up-to-date representation of the knowledge about a particular subject. The use of systems as an electronic textbook may prove more important at a practical level than their use for decision-support (Heath-field & Wyatt 1993).

Sharing knowledge bases

No one group can develop a knowledge base embracing the whole of medicine. In order that the products of different groups can be shared it is essential that standards be developed. An initiative towards such standards (the Arden Syntax; Hripesak et al. 1991) has already begun.

Domain-independent CMD systems (expert systems shells)

Most well-known CMD systems were originally described for a specific application, e.g. MYCIN for antibiotic therapy. Some were further developed into so-called expert system shells or domain-independent systems which provide all the relevant software tools and then allow the user to construct an application – in effect, to write the knowledge base. Shells might be the quickest and easiest way of developing an expert system, but they are expensive, slow, and can leave the user with little control over the finished product (Schreiner & Chard 1990).

There are numerous commercially available 'shells' which could be used for medical applications. The choice between these products is extraordinarily confusing (Ellis 1987). In addition, certain high-level languages have been advocated for use in expert systems, notably PROLOG and LISP. But it is interesting to note that current implementation of two classical LISP-based systems, PUFF and Internist, are now written in BASIC and Pascal respectively. Furthermore, medical applications often require an extensive database. Database facilities on expert system shells are often limited: it may be simpler to add inferencing facilities to a database than to add a database to the shell.

Some general rules for the design of CMD systems

Regardless of which approach or approaches is adopted, there are certain pragmatic rules which should guide the development of any CMD system:

1. The system should at least attempt to find a single diagnosis which accounts for all the data (the principle known as Occam's razor).
2. At the same time, the system should be capable of partitioning if it is apparent that there is more than one diagnosis.
3. The system should proceed from the general to the specific, i.e. having identified the broad area of a problem it should focus on smaller subsets.
4. The system should be capable of eliminating a diagnosis; this is often simpler than making a diagnosis and can be just as helpful.
5. The items of information which have the greatest differential diagnostic value should be sought first.

6. The system should recognise that common events are common, and that a massive and encyclopaedic list of differential diagnoses can be counter-productive.
7. The system should never miss a treatable disease.
8. The system should never leave important factors unexplained.

At a strictly practical level, Heathfield & Wyatt (1993) have very usefully pointed out that 'the effort involved in developing, maintaining and supporting ... a decision support system ... is often severely underestimated'.

Presenting the findings of a CMD system

There is much variation in the format for presentation of the conclusions of a CMD system. Options range from the simple to the complex. The simplest system presents only the most likely diagnosis. At the other extreme the machine can present a complete list of rank-ordered diagnoses, together with the exact probabilities of each and a formal statement of the factors which were taken into consideration in reaching these conclusions. In between are systems which present a diagnosis or diagnoses classified simply as probable or possible. The latter more closely emulate the normal human process and are therefore likely to be the most favoured. Svenmondt & Cooper (1993) have shown that providing explanations of inference results can enhance diagnostic accuracy in a decision-support system for anaesthesia.

Performance assessment of a CMD system

Each of the CMD systems described above has its own band of dedicated and enthusiastic supporters. However, studies which attempt to compare the performance of different CMD systems seem to agree that there is little to choose between them (reviewed by Reggia and Tuhrim 1985). The latter authors present the very wise counsel that methods should be chosen according to the specific problem: in particular, in accordance with the format in which the knowledge is already encoded. For example, there are several well-documented sets of clinical rules which lend themselves well to the knowledge base of a production rule system and which can therefore be used with very little 'translation'. Similarly, there are some problems which demand a probabilistic solution of the Bayesian type (for example prognosis of strokes or heart attacks) while others involve categorical inferences (for example staging of cancer). Systems which combine a number of different approaches are probably the optimum.

Formal critical assessment of CMD systems is still very limited in scope (reviewed by Weaver 1991; Wyatt & Spiegelhalter 1992; Langton et al. 1993). The criteria for assessment of any CMD system should be accuracy, usefulness, transferability and acceptability.

Table 5.4. The definitions of true and false positives, and true and false negatives

True positive (TP):	The result is positive in the presence of the clinical abnormality
True negative (TN):	The result is negative in the absence of the clinical abnormality
False positive (FP):	The result is positive in the absence of the clinical abnormality
False negative (FN):	The result is negative in the presence of the clinical abnormality

Table 5.5. The definitions of sensitivity, specificity and predictive value

Sensitivity	$\dfrac{TP}{(TP + FN)}$	$\dfrac{5}{(5 + 5)}$	$= 50\%$
Specificity	$\dfrac{TN}{(FP + TN)}$	$\dfrac{85}{(5 + 85)}$	$= 94.4\%$
Predictive value	$\dfrac{TP}{(FP + TP)}$	$\dfrac{5}{(5 + 5)}$	$= 50\%$

TP, TN etc are defined in Table 5.4. The numbers given are from a hypothetical study involving a population of 100 patients, 10 of whom have disease X. The diagnostic system correctly identifies five of these cases (true positives) misses five cases (false negatives) and makes an incorrect diagnosis in five cases (false positives).

Accuracy

The accuracy (or efficiency) of any diagnostic system is assessed by determining the rates of true and false positive results, and true and false negatives (defined in Table 5.4). From these the sensitivity, specificity and predictive value are calculated as shown in Table 5.5. Put in words, sensitivity is an index of the proportion of all cases of the clinical abnormality correctly identified by the system; specificity is an index of the proportion of all patients in whom the absence of the condition is correctly identified; predictive value is an index of the proportion of all patients in whom the condition is identified by the system and who actually have the condition.

Once estimated, the sensitivity, specificity and predictive value of a CMD system in respect of a given diagnosis are compared with the figures derived from some 'gold standard' of correctness. Typically this would be the conclusion reached by an expert physician given the same information. One problem of this type of comparison is that the CMD system is likely to reach a conclusion based on exact probability whereas the physician's conclusion will be qualitative. The machine may decide that diagnosis X is correct because it has a probability of 0.75 whereas the next most likely diagnosis, Y, has a probability of 0.5. A human may reach the same conclusion, but it will be in the form 'X is the most likely diagnosis and Y is the next most likely', i.e. without any estimate of the closeness of the probabilities. In addition, humans tend to be more confident about the accuracy of their guesses than is justified by the real probabilities. Humans also tend to ignore negative information in favour of positive facts which confirm their hypotheses.

CMD systems can also be compared among themselves by comparison of the probabilities reached in respect of conditions for which there is some absolute measure of outcome. Take, for example, a brain tumour. The final arbiter of this diagnosis will be the histology of a surgical specimen. However, all the information obtained prior to surgery can be combined in a CMD system. If one system gave probability 0.8 in the actual presence of a tumour while another system gave 0.6, then clearly the first system is more 'correct' than the second. This is not the end of the story, of course, because the first system might give large numbers of false positives which would indicate unnecessary surgery.

The design and implementation of studies which compare humans with CMD systems can be fraught with problems. Notable among these is the 'study paradox': the introduction of structured data collection forms, essential for the comparison, will often enhance diagnostic accuracy without the use of the computer (Hancock et al. 1987; Lilford et al. 1992).

Despite this there have been many studies in which the accuracy of machine diagnosis has been compared with that of a human faced with the same data. Generally the machine is equivalent or somewhat superior to the human. The best known of such comparisons, that of de Dombal et al. (1972) on abdominal pain, is described below. Other examples include jaundice (Malchow-Moller et al. 1986; Camma et al. 1991), genital infections (Chard 1987b), acid–base balance (Schrenck et al. 1986), head injury (the Glasgow Coma Scale; Barlow et al. 1987), critical care (Chang et al. 1989), myocardial infarction (Goldman et al. 1988; Gilpin et al. 1990), trauma (Clarke et al. 1988) and electrocardiography (Willems et al. 1991). The machine is especially strong in expert systems involving simple but multiple calculations. With acid–base balance, for instance, machine and human are nearly equivalent as regards single disorders, but human performance deteriorates sharply where there are triple disorders (Schrenck et al. 1986). In general, machines are less likely to make false positive predictions than humans (e.g. McNutt & Selker 1988; Chang et al. 1989). Not surprisingly, performance also varies between different programs, a fact well documented in the case of electrocardiography (Willems et al. 1991).

Usefulness

To be successful a CMD system must offer some advantage over humans. Machines and the best human experts are equivalent in terms of accuracy. But the real advantage of the machine is that it may be available when the human expert is not, and under these circumstances there can be no doubt as to usefulness. A notable example is the use of the de Dombal abdominal pain system in US navy submarines (Henderson and Black 1980). On a mission these can receive but not send messages. The use of a CMD system can provide powerful reassurance to isolated medical corpsmen and obviate the danger and cost of surfacing unnecessarily. Similar systems have been devised by NASA for use by isolated astronauts on space missions (Grams & Jin 1989). However, it must not always be assumed that accuracy and acceptability equate to usefulness. In a controlled study on an advisory system for chest pain, Wyatt (1989) has shown that a system which performs well in the laboratory may fail to alter the clinical management of patients.

Other practical factors which may be looked for in a CMD system include:

1. *Speed.* A system will be of no value if it takes several minutes to digest or divulge a piece of information.
2. *Authority.* The system must reflect widely accepted views on a topic, not the idiosyncrasies of a particular designer. This is not a problem when, as at present, most systems are at a prototype stage; however, it is likely to become so when the subject matures and multiple competing systems are available. This is the current situation with computer-based interpretation of psychological tests, a topic which has been active since the 1950s (Hofer & Green 1985; Moreland 1985). Another problem is that experts may reach the same conclusion by different routes, as shown in a study by Gilpin et al. (1990) on predictive outcome following myocardial infarction.
3. *Cost.* CMD system will usually be an addition to other medical expenses, but can generate savings through greater efficiency. For example, giving physicians predicted probabilities of test abnormalities and costs for commonly ordered laboratory tests can yield a significant reduction in patient charges (Tierney et al. 1988, 1990). A reduction in the need for patient admission has been shown with the use of CMD for abdominal pain (Adams et al. 1986) and myocardial infarction (Goldman et al. 1988).

Transferability

Will a CMD system work on a site other than that where it originated, and with different staff? A database for symptoms and signs of jaundice developed at a specialised liver unit in London (Knill-Jones et al. 1973) was shown to be inadequate for use in a Swedish hospital (Lindberg 1982). However, a later study showed that another jaundice algorithm, this time developed in Copenhagen, worked well in a Swedish setting (Lindberg et al. 1987). In the UK, transferability has been clearly demonstrated for the de Dombal system for abdominal pain.

Acceptability

The introduction of a CMD system may be seen by some healthcare personnel, notably physicians, as an intrusion upon their professional domain and standing. It has even been suggested that computerised diagnostic aids are less welcome when services are reimbursed on a fee-per-item basis than in free or pre-paid healthcare plans (Kleinmuntz & Elstein, 1987). However, professional objections are usually short-lived: the image of the physician may even be enhanced by his use of sophisticated technology. At an introductory stage, CMD systems should always be advocated for decision support rather than decision making.

Another objection is that the use of a CMD system may add steps (and therefore time) to the diagnosis process. This is the case with many current CMD systems, including those of the de Dombal group, which are independent of the data collection process, i.e. selected data are transferred to the system after completion of the encounter with the patient. The need for double entry must be regarded as a constraint. In the more successful systems, such as that at the Beth Israel Hospital in Boston, the decision support functions are closely integrated with clinical data CMD systems (laboratory reports etc.) (Bleich et al. 1989; Safran et al. 1990).

Some examples of a CMD system in action

Examples of expert diagnostic systems in specific clinical areas are listed in Table 5.6. Some of the better-known systems will be reviewed in more detail here.

Table 5.6. Some published examples of the use of expert systems in particular areas of diagnosis. Maceratini and colleagues (1989) have provided a very detailed review of this area

Abdominal pain	Adams et al. 1986; Fenyo 1990
Emergency triage	Berman et al. 1989
Trauma	Clarke et al. 1988
Chest pain	Goldman et al. 1988; Kennedy et al. 1993
Jaundice	Lindberg et al. 1987
Acid–base balance	Schrenck et al. 1986
Gynaecological endocrinology	Schreiner & Chard 1990
Primary healthcare	Gordon 1991
Low back pain	Mann & Brown 1991
Neonatal heart disease	Franklin et al. 1991
Electrocardiology	Willems et al. 1991
Rheumatic diseases	Moens & Korst 1992
Stroke	Wain et al. 1992
Psychiatry	First et al. 1993

INTERNIST (Caduceus)

INTERNIST is the best known of the systems said to be based on a cognitive model (Miller et al. 1986). The knowledge base includes about 575 diseases and more than 4000 individual manifestations of disease (demographics, history, symptoms, physical signs and laboratory data). The knowledge base consists of profiles of diseases. All the manifestations of the disease are listed and three numbers are assigned to each manifestation, each on a scale from 1 to 5. The first number ('evoking strength') addresses the question, 'On the basis of this finding alone, how strongly does the physician consider the patient has this disease compared with any other in internal medicine?' The second number ('frequency') states that, given the disease, the manifestation occurs with a certain frequency (1 = rare or minimal; 2 = a significant minority of cases; 3 = about half of the cases; 4 = a significant majority of cases; and 5 = essentially all). Each manifestation is given a third number ('importance') indicating whether it is necessary to explain the manifestation in presenting the diagnosis.

The inference engine of INTERNIST-1 considers each disease which is compatible with any positive manifestation on the basis of the evoking strength numbers. Positive manifestations will therefore cluster in the most probable diagnoses. The values for each of the three numbers permit ranking of the diagnoses evoked. If the leading contender has adequate support, this is concluded as the diagnosis. If it does not, the system asks for additional observations.

A later development from INTERNIST-1 is the QUICK MEDICAL REFERENCE program (QMR) (Miller et al. 1986). This relies on the same knowledge base, but whereas INTERNIST-1 is a diagnostic consultant, QMR acts as an information tool so that users can review the knowledge base. It is available for microcomputers and has been very well received by users (Bankowitz et al. 1989). Providing an 'electronic textbook' of this type is one of the most important real-life practical functions of many expert systems (Wyatt 1991).

The de Dombal system for abdominal pain

de Dombal and colleagues in Leeds have been pioneers of the practical application of expert systems in medicine. In 1972 they described a program for the diagnosis of acute abdominal pain (de Dombal et al. 1972) and since then have published regular improvements and updates. The most recent of these (Adams et al. 1986) is worth reviewing because it is a model of how such systems should be designed and evaluated.

The program was designed for the evaluation of cases of abdominal pain of less than 1 week's duration presenting at a hospital emergency department. The information from each patient is compared, using a

Bayesian probabilistic analysis, with reference data derived from 6000 patients in 13 countries.

The system was evaluated in eight centres with more than 250 participating doctors and 16 737 patients. Performance in respect of diagnosis and decision-making was compared over a baseline period with no computer assistance and a test period with the machine system. The results were extraordinarily impressive. Initial diagnostic accuracy rose from 45.6 per cent to 65.3 per cent. The rate of negative laparotomies fell by half, as did the rate of perforation in patients with appendicitis. Serious management errors fell from 0.9 per cent to 0.2 per cent and mortality by 22 per cent. It was estimated that savings were made by the avoidance of 278 laparotomies and 8516 bed nights during the trial period. A study such as this leaves little doubt that CMD systems must play an increasing role in the practice of clinical medicine.

Possibly because of its success the de Dombal system has come in for some criticism. For example, Sutton (1989) has attributed the improvement in patient management to structured data collection and audit feedback rather than any merits in the Bayesian diagnostic system itself. While there may be some measure of truth in this, the alternative explanation still constitutes a powerful argument for the use of systems of this type.

DXplain

DXplain is one of the latest and most practical of diagnostic decision-support systems, developed at Massachussetts General Hospital in collaboration with the American Medical Association (Barnett et al. 1987). The system is distributed through AMA/NET and thus is available to anyone with a terminal and modem. The knowledge base consists of descriptions of approximately 2000 diseases, about 4700 terms (signs, symptoms, etc.), and some 65 000 relationships among them. These items are linked by relatively straightforward algorithms and selection rules based on a scoring system similar to a Bayesian computation. Thus the system acts very much as an 'electronic textbook', providing fast and easy access to medical knowledge. The physician inputs clinical findings and the system produces a list of ordered diagnostic hypotheses, if necessary with explanations and requests for additional facts. An important feature is the collaboration with users, whose comments and suggestions are continuously reviewed in order to modify and enhance the knowledge base.

The multi-centre Chest Pain Study

The multi-centre Chest Pain Study prospectively evaluated 4770 patients presenting with acute chest pain (Goldman et al. 1988). The computer protocol had a higher specificity (ability to predict absence of infarction) than physicians and a similar sensitivity (ability to detect presence of infarction). Decisions based on computer protocols alone would have reduced admission of patients without infarction by 11.5 per cent while not affecting admission of patients who required intensive care. In other words, the computer corrects the tendency for the physician to over-estimate risk in cases with a low probability of acute ischaemia (McNutt & Selker 1988). The system can also reduce (from 24 to 12 hours) the observation period needed to exclude myocardial infarction (Lee et al. 1991).

Self-diagnosis and self-treatment

There are numerous programs available for use on home computers which provide advice on medical matters. Some of these offer simple diagnostic algorithms for common symptoms; others provide specific guidelines for diet, life-style, etc. The extent of the likely use of such programs, as with home computers themselves, has probably been some-what exaggerated.

Legal aspects of CMD systems

CMD systems, alone or when used by skilled personnel, have the potential to injure patients. The computer might suggest an incorrect diagnosis, or miss a potentially dangerous drug interaction, or fail to call for necessary treatment. One widely quoted example is that of a radio-therapy machine in Texas which had two modes: a normal therapeutic mode and a research mode which allowed an unobstructed high-intensity X-ray beam to travel through the accelerator guide, destroying all tissues in its path. Two patients were alleged to have died as a result of failure of software to switch between these modes (Joyce 1987). Inevitably, the question of liability for a computer program will result in a lawsuit and the implications for this in the US have been reviewed in detail (Brannigan & Mola 1990). The main issues are whether a program is a product or a service, and whether an error will be attributed to the designers or to the producers.

Is the program a product or a service?

If programs are considered as products, then manufacturers and distribu-tors will be held to a strict product liability standard. If programs are considered as services, then the producers and users will be liable only if they can be shown to be negligent (fault liability). Medical computer programs do not fall neatly into either category, but in both the US and

Europe* it seems like that the standard of strict liability will apply. In other words, the legal system will impose liability on the computer which it would not impose on the physician.

Is a program error a design defect or a production defect?

If the error is considered to be in the design of a program, then liability can only be assessed after review of the possibility of alternative designs. Furthermore, a court might have to decide which of the many 'creators' of a program might have been responsible for the plaintiff's 'injury'. If the defect is in production, then liability exists even if due care had been exercised in the production process.

Who will be sued and on what grounds?

In any case involving software liability there are three potential defendants: the individual clinician, the hospital and the software manufacturer. For a variety of legal and commercial reasons it would appear that the physician will probably not be held liable and that the software manufacturer is the most likely target. A case against a software manufacturer might be based on a breach of express warranty, breach of implied warranties, negligence or strict product liability. The latter is the most demanding because liability exists even if there was no fault on the part of the producer; however, it seems that this is the most likely standard. Software manufacturers will seek to protect themselves against claims by a combination of disclaimers, restriction of liability, indemnities by users and insurance.

Regulation of medical computer software

In the US it is probable that federal regulators will control medical computer software as a 'device' under the Food, Drug and Cosmetic Act (FDCA) (Brannigan 1987; Murfitt 1990; Furfine 1992; Gammerman 1992).† Similar arrangements may apply in Europe. If clinical systems are controlled, they will be in either class II (which includes most diagnostic equipment) or class III (which includes therapeutic equipment such as pacemakers). The demands of class III are very stringent including pre-market approval based on appropriate testing. The problems of definition are considerable because software is intangible and conveys ideas rather than direct effects; if software is considered as 'ideas' then it may be

---

* EC Product Liability Directive (85/374/EEC).

† More detailed guidance can be obtained from the Division of Small Manufacturers Assistance, Center for Devices and Radiological Health (HFZ-220), 5600 Fishers Lane, Rockville, MD 20857, USA.

protected from regulation by the First Amendment of the Constitution (freedom of the Press). Furthermore, it is difficult to distinguish manufacturing, which is federally regulated, from use, which is State regulated. Brannigan (1987) has stated 'public interest would be best served ... by modest regulation on the user ... providing a mix of consumer protection with minimum restriction on ... this revolutionary technology'.

Conclusions

Some degree of computer assistance with medical diagnosis is certain to grow – especially as part of computerised clinical data collection systems. Reasons for this growth include the increasing complexity of the medical knowledge base, the increasing specialisation of medical practice, the increasing availability of powerful computer technology, and increasing willingness of physicians to make use of computer technology. However, CMD systems must always be seen as supporting and not in any way replacing the physician's own decision-making process; the term 'cognitive prosthesis' has been very aptly used to describe the use of computers to augment human intellect. CMD systems must be readily accessible, easy to use, and authoritative. It is the failure of most prototype systems to meet these obvious criteria which explains why CMD systems are not already an integral part of routine medical care. To paraphrase Shortliffe (1991) 'Physicians will be attracted to computers when they are useful ... for every patient they see, and when ... system use is consistent across varied applications ... the limited success of knowledge-based systems is ... due more to failure of integration than ... to any basic problem with A1 technologies'.

6

Computers and treatment

Computers have many actual and potential uses in medical treatment. Areas in which they are particularly successful include radiotherapy and critical care. Indeed, there are procedures which would not be possible at all without computer assistance.

Introduction

There is often only a narrow gap between procedures which can be described as 'diagnosis' and those which can be described as 'treatment'. Thus the diagnosis of an infection will commonly lead to the prescription of an antibiotic: this is a small, straightforward and logical step which can readily be performed by a machine and therefore constitutes an example of treatment by computer. Furthermore, it presents no problem if there are numerous caveats to the decision such as enquiry about patient allergy, previous therapy, age of patient, other current medication etc. Indeed, the rigorous exploration of possible contraindications to the line of management is a task to which the computer is particularly well-suited.

There are many examples of the use of computers as part of patient treatment. Some have already been addressed (e.g. the use of computers in a hospital pharmacy). Here some general uses of computers in medical treatment will be discussed together with specific applications in selected areas.

The use of computers to prompt medical action

McDonald (1976) pointed out that the commonest reason for errors or mistakes in medical care is oversight rather than ignorance. He suggested that this was due to intrinsic human limits on information processing, especially as regards simple but very repetitive tasks. Since then many protocols have been devised which provide reminders and action suggestions, often built into data collection systems. A typical protocol might remind the physician to check the serum potassium at least once a year in patients on thiazide diuretics; the protocol could also suggest action in the event of an abnormal result.

Medical prompts have been divided into two types: cueing and monitoring (Friedman 1986). Cueing is prospective: taking the example above, the physician would automatically be alerted to order a serum potassium test each year. Monitoring is retrospective: the physician would be alerted if, after one year, no potassium determination had been carried out. An example of monitoring is the CARE system described by McDonald et al. (1984) which monitors on-line medical records and sends reminders when a laboratory result should be checked. The benefits of such prompts have been well documented by a computerised laboratory alerting system which showed substantial improvement in the clinical response to situations such as low potassium levels (Tate et al. 1990). The balance between cueing and monitoring is very much a matter of style. An excess of cues, covering every possible decision, can be unwelcome to the physician; under many circumstances monitoring is preferable. At the same time, cues are essential for decisions which must be made before the event; for example, a history of iodine sensitivity must be established before and not after an intravenous pyelogram. In practice, cueing and monitoring are often combined in the same system.

An example of a system which combines clinical data collection with management protocols is the Cancer Data Management System (CDMS) developed at Boston University School of Medicine (Friedman 1986). The basis of this is a structured data collection system, coupled to a library of information on therapeutic agents and treatment plans. Therapy selection is assisted by matching characteristics of the patient with information in the CDMS regarding indications and contraindications (Table 6.1). The same type of advisory process can be applied to each step of the recursive process which Friedman (1986) has referred to as the 'medical management loop' (Fig. 6.1).

Critiquing

Critiquing is the name given to a monitoring system in which the physician indicates his or her planned management and the machine responds with the advantages and disadvantages of the proposed approach together with suggestions for alternatives (Miller 1986). Because a critiquing model demands a complex dialogue, such systems are awkward to build and are presently only available in prototype form.

The use of computers for surveillance of medical action

The computerised treatment record can be used for high-level surveillance of management protocols. This approach is now widely used for research, peer review and administrative purposes. A notable example with a positive outcome is a system for the evaluation of work-related back injuries (Wiesal & Michelson 1986). If the patient's diagnosis,

Table 6.1. An example of a prompt system to check possible treatment options for a patient with cancer (modified from the CDMS system described by Friedman 1986)

Patient: JX   IDNo 123456   Date: 10.2.87
Patient information needed
Activity status of patient

1.   Normal activities
2.   Symptomatic but ambulatory
3.   Confined to bed less than 50 per cent
4.   Confined to bed more than 50 per cent
5.   100 per cent bedridden

Activity status? [2]   [Date? 10.2.87]

White blood count? [4.8]   [Date?   8.2.87]

Platelet count? [350]   [Date?   8.2.87]

Serum creatinine? [not done]

Regimen advised
CDV (Cyclophosphamide, doxorubicin, vincristine)
   The patient is eligible for this protocol

Alternative regimen
CED (Cyclophosphamide, etoposide, cis-platinum)
   The patient may be eligible for this protocol
   Check the following:
      Serum creatinine

Information of this type is available as a computerised databank: the Patient Data Query system organised by the National Cancer Institute. This can be accessed by dialling into the MEDLARS system.

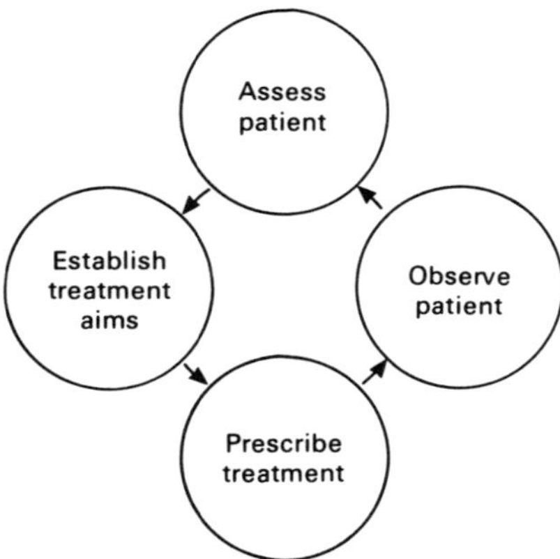

Fig. 6.1. The 'medical management loop'. This shows the sequence of decisions which physicians make in patient treatment; the loop may be repeated many times. Each part of the loop can be the subject of a computer advisory system of the type shown in Table 6.1. Cancer chemotherapy lends itself particularly well to this type of therapeutic expert system.

treatment or clinical progress differ from that predicted by the computer, an independent medical examination is obtained. This system was evaluated for one year on 14 000 employees in the US Postal Service. There was a 41 per cent decrease in days lost from work, and a 55 per cent decrease in costs.

The use of computers for surveillance of screening programmes

There are many familiar examples of population screening programmes in which there is little doubt about the efficiency of the procedure, and for which success is judged by the percentage of the target population who receive the test. Examples include neonatal screening for phenylketonuria (PKU) and congenital hypothyroidism (CHT; Meaney 1988), and cervical cytology. A study of prompting for preventive procedures in general practice showed a notable advantage to a computer system (no prompts 38%; nurse prompts 43%; computer prompts 53%; Harris et al. 1990). The gain was most notable with influenza vaccination and mammography, less so for faecal blood testing and cervical cytology. It is often possible to link a computer in the department providing the service with another containing a database of the complete population. Thus, in the UK, linkage of laboratory computers to the universal child-health computer system has had a dramatic impact on the penetration of PKU and CHT testing (Griffiths et al. 1987). In the US, progress in the use of computers for tracking newborn screening and follow-up has been less satisfactory (Meaney 1988).

Decision analysis

In many treatment situations the decision-making process departs radically from simple one-to-one logic. Traditionally this is dealt with by 'intuition' (some would say guesswork). But in recent years there have been many attempts to quantitate the process of 'difficult' decision making, and a whole new subject has emerged which is referred to as decision analysis. Computers have played an important part in both the development and application of this subject.*

Decision analysis involves identifying all possible management choices (the 'strategies'), estimating the potential outcomes of each choice, and then preparing a model, usually in the form of a decision 'tree' (Fig. 6.2). Each decision point in the tree is a 'node'. The relative worth, or 'utility', of each outcome is quantitated on a numeric scale: an example might be 0 for immediate death running to 100 for normal life expectancy. The most

---

* A decision analysis program for the IBM PC (Decision Maker 5.3) is available from Dr S Pauker, New England Medical Center, 171 Harrison Avenue, Boston, MA 02111, USA.

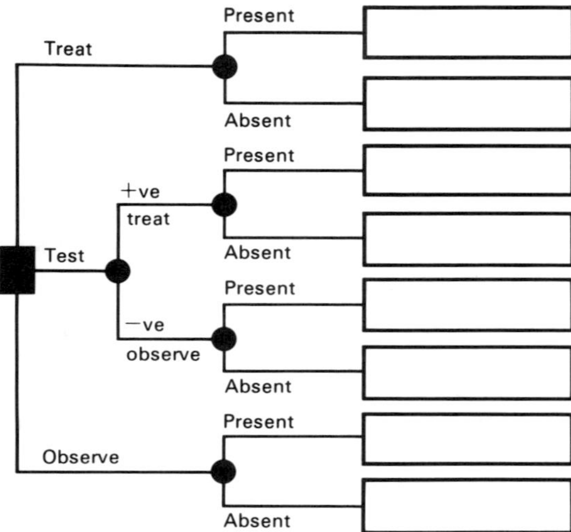

Fig. 6.2. A schematic of a decision tree. The square node on the left denotes a point in the clinical process at which a decision has to be made; either to treat immediately, or to perform a further test before deciding, or to do nothing. Most decisions in medicine can be reduced to this, 'treat, test, observe' paradigm. The circular nodes denote chance points, depicting events determined by probability. The rectangular terminal nodes denote the outcome.

rational course of action is the strategy with maximal utility. One of the techniques of decision analysis which lends itself to computation is sensitivity analysis. This is a 'what if' exercise in which the variable is changed to determine whether it affects the decision. When drawn as a graph this may show an intersection of strategy lines, often referred to as decision thresholds. A threshold is the probability above which one management strategy is optimal and below which another is optimal (Kassirer et al. 1987; Pauker & Kassirer 1987).

With a few notable exceptions decision analysis is of limited usefulness. As with computerised medical diagnosis, the estimation of utility depends on a substantial database which may not always be available. Furthermore, the perception of risk is a very subjective phenomenon. Concepts of probability are hard to grasp, even for experienced physicians (Slovic 1987; Wilson & Crouch 1987). Humans do not use the same global process as a machine in reaching decisions but rather a 'chain ... together with a sequence of decisions based on ... incomplete information' (Moskowitz et al. 1988). In an attempt to solve this problem, systems have been described which automatically convert numerical probability data into a combination of diagrams and English language (Langlotz et al. 1988). An additional element of randomness is introduced by the fact that more than one party is usually involved in the decision: contributors may include the doctor, the patient, and providers of healthcare resources. For this reason it has been seriously proposed that medical decision analysis should be regarded as a branch of game-theory (Diamond et al. 1986).

The use of computers in specific areas of medical treatment

There are many examples of the use of computers in specific medical situations. Some of these are listed in Table 6.2 and discussed further below.

Table 6.2. Some published examples of the use of computers in specific patient care situations

Situation	Reference
Critical care (fluid balance, respiratory and cardiovascular function)	Siegel & Coleman 1986
Craniofacial surgery	Cutting et al. 1986; Salyer et al. 1986
Orthopaedic surgery	Pho et al. 1990; Goh et al. 1990
Anaesthesia	Prakash 1983
Optimising drug dosage:	
Antibiotics	Lenert et al. 1992
Digoxin	Crevasse et al. 1988
Anticoagulants and thrombolysis	White (1987); Kellett & O'Riordon 1992
Lidocaine	Vozeh 1987
Insulin	Saudek et al. 1989; Peterson et al. 1986; Hauser et al. 1992
Therapy for depression	Selmi et al. 1991
Total parenteral nutrition	Shami 1986; Legler 1990
Alcoholism	Meier & Sampson 1989
Sex therapy	Binik et al. 1989; Alemi et al. 1989
Radiotherapy	Wong & Chua 1990
Smoking abstinence	Schneider et al. 1990
Asthma	(Osman et al. 1994)
Health crisis management	(Gustafson et al. 1993)

Radiotherapy

Radiotherapy is one area of treatment which could no longer be practised without computers. The uses include treatment planning, dose calculations, localisation of tumours, verification of patient set-ups and radiation beam data acquisition (reviewed by Wong & Chua 1990). Radiotherapy was also the subject of the only serious medical disaster attributable to computers: the 'Therac-25' incident in which a software fault led to gross overdoses (Jacky 1989).

Critical care

For many intensive therapy situations the rapid analysis of complex data is so important that it must be regarded as part of the treatment process. Such situations include fluid balance and respiratory and cardiovascular function (Prakash 1983; Siegel & Coleman 1986). Specific packages have been devised for these purposes, a well-known example being the Patient Data Management System (PDMS) developed by Hewlett-Packard in the late 1970s; this package automates a variety of charting functions normally performed by nursing, laboratory and other ancillary services. Monitoring systems of this type can compare current findings with predetermined criteria and activate alarm systems if appropriate.* Furthermore, some systems can provide automatic intervention to correct detected abnormalities. Examples include administration of medications, changes in ventilator settings, and adjustments of intravenous flow-rates.

Anaesthesia

Computers have a wide variety of actual or potential applications in anaesthesia (Prakash 1983) most of which are data collection and data analysis functions similar to those in other specialties. More specific systems are systems which integrate the administration of intravenous agents and the response to such agents (reviewed by O'Hara et al. 1992). Published examples include the use of sodium nitroprusside for the management of hypertensive crises in the postoperative cardiac patient (Pace & Westenskow 1983), and the automatic control of infusion of muscle relaxants and narcotics (Ritchie et al 1983). Such systems add a 'fly by wire' dimension to the subject which would not be available from the traditional manual approach. In other words, the availability of fast, automatic feedback ('automatic closed loop control') (Evans et al. 1983) allows formats of administration which would not be possible with manual techniques.

Prescribing

Computers are now widely used in the prescribing of drugs. An inexpensive personal computer system (RxWRITER) is available from Hall Design Inc., 250 Maple Avenue, Wilmette, IL 60091, USA. This can go well beyond simple wordprocessing functions (Fig. 6.3).

---

* Messages delivered by a tape-recorded human voice are more effective than non-verbal signals (McIntyre & Nelson 1991).

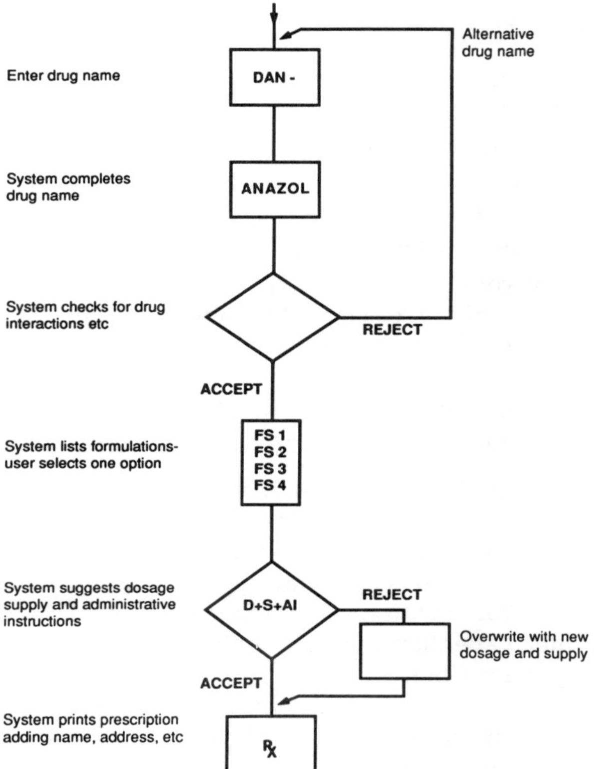

Fig 6.3. A computerised prescribing system

There are a number of situations in which the therapeutic dose of a drug is very close to the toxic dose. Under these circumstances great care has to be taken in designing dosage schedules and the effects are often monitored by measurement of circulating levels. Notable examples include digoxin, antiarrhythmics, aminoglycoside antibiotics, and anti-coagulants. A computer can be of great assistance in the complex decisions involved; a number of such programs have been described both specific (Table 6.2) and generalised (Proost & Meijer 1992). Computer-generated reminders can be of great value in ensuring compliance (Raynor et al. 1993; Osman et al. 1994).

Handicap

One of the most dramatic applications of computers is their use in improving the lifestyle of handicapped patients.*

---

* Some of the most remarkable devices are amusingly reviewed by Rochester & Gantz in the *Naked Computer* (Arlington Books, 1983).

Deafness and speechlessness

A number of devices are under development to aid the deaf and speech-less. These include:

1. An artificial cochlea (the connection between the inner ear and the auditory nerve). Auditory signals are produced by computer and input via electrodes attached to selected locations along the cochlea (Blamey et al. 1987; Schindler et al. 1993).
2. The tactual vocoder, a non-invasive device that transforms acoustic energy into vibratory electrotactile sensations on the user's skin (Blamey & Clark 1987). The best of these are now equivalent to the cochlea implant.
3. A device which enables the keypad of any telephone to be used to transmit characters to a VDU at the receiving point.

The problems of teaching hearing-impaired children to read and write have been reviewed in detail by Prinz et al. (1985). These authors have developed an interactive microcomputer system (named ALPHA) in which pictures, text and sign language are directly initiated by the children via a keyboard with specially made word overlays. The system is particularly aimed at enhancing communication with the teacher, rather than replacing the teacher.

Some systems are of extraordinary ingenuity. For example, deaf–blind persons can sometimes receive speech by placing a hand on the face of the talker and monitoring facial actions associated with speech (the Tadoma method). There is now a synthetic Tadoma system which a computer-driven artificial face (Leotta et al. 1988).

Blindness

Various devices to aid the visually impaired have been described (reviewed by Boulton 1993). Computer-based reading systems which automatically translate print into speech are available,* as are audio-typing units which produce sounds corresponding to typewriter keys. Attempts have been made to convey graphical information to the blind via various tactile devices such as the use of 'sound graphs' in which a continuously varying pitch is used to represent motion into the horizontal direction (Mansur et al. 1985). Work towards artificial vision has been described which uses a matrix for electrodes implanted on a blind person's visual cortex. The electrodes can be wired to appropriate devices (miniature TV cameras) on the outside of the skull.

---

* For example, PC Voice from ARTS Computer Productions Inc, 145 Tremont Street, Suite 407, Boston, MA 02111, USA.

Electrical stimulation of paralysed muscles

Several microprocessor controlled functions for the electrical stimulation of paralysed muscles are being evaluated:

1. Stimulation sequences for electrodes implanted into specific muscle groups in paraplegics.
2. Combinations of sensors and stimulators which enable the posture of the upper body to produce actions in the lower limbs.
3. A system for restoring bladder control via electrodes placed surgically in the roots of the sacral nerves: the electrodes can respond to a radio signal.
4. Computer-driven prostheses: the most effective way for controlling a powered arm prosthesis is the use of electromyographic (EMG) signals from the user. Muscles still present on the proximal aspect of the arm are used to control the distal artificial arm.

Cognitive rehabilitation of brain-injured persons

Survivors of strokes, intracranial tumours and head injuries may suffer impairment of higher cognitive processes such as memory, problem-solving, visual–spatial skills, and language. Computers can now play an important part both in the assessment and the retraining of these functions (Kurlychek & Levin 1988).

Devices which enable the disabled to control their environment

The ability to use a computer for communication and other purposes can provide an extra dimension to the life of the handicapped. Disabled persons often cannot manipulate a standard keyboard. Devices which provide assistance include touch-screens, light pens, joysticks, voice volume and pitch detectors, mouth sticks, foot operated switches and the ubiquitous 'mouse'. Of particular importance is the so-called scanning keyboard (Treviranus & Tannock 1987). This is a screen access which a cursor travels in a preset pattern. The user activates a switch which can stop the cursor at any desired item. The switch can be activated by the simplest of voluntary movements, for example the pneumatic puff–sip devices or eye movement devices (Kilgallon et al. 1987)* used by many high level quadriplegics. Computer devices are now available which permit the disabled to control most of the standard domestic environment (Dickey & Shealey 1987). This includes lighting and heating, radio and TV, kitchen equipment, bed controls, page turners, door locks and other security devices.

---

* The Eyegaze System (LC Technologies Inc, 4415 Glenn Rose Street, Faifax, VA 22032, USA).

Devices to supervise the mentally handicapped

A computer assisted program has been described for promoting the performance of unsupervised activities by adolescents with multiple impairment (Lancioni & Oliva 1988). Although this approach has been criticised as an attempt to reduce staff–patient interaction, it would be of great value in institutions where direct supervision is not possible for large parts of the day.

Reconstructive surgery

The planning of craniofacial surgery has always been an artistic rather than a scientific endeavour. However, computers have been used to generate and manipulate images from measurements obtained by encephalography, cephalometry, multiple thin-slice tocography and standard photographs of the face (Cutting et al. 1986; Marsh et al. 1986; Salyer et al. 1986). The procedure by which a computer makes and manipulates models of objects is quite different from that of simply presenting an image. The latter is 'pixel-based' and the end result is essentially a static digital description. Modelling, by contrast, requires an 'object-based' approach. A circle, for example, is stored as the coordinates of its centre plus the radius. The image can then be manipulated mathematically – the sort of system already widely used in industrial design.

Reconstruction can be performed by dividing the object space into 3-D volume elements called 'voxels' (analogous to 'pixels'). This demands very large amounts of storage for an adequate presentation (as for example Control Data's ICEM solid modeller, West & Skytte 1985). Presentation as a true three-dimensional display also requires specialised hardware such as varifocal mirror, stereoscopic apparatus or holography, which is impractical for most clinical purposes. Consequently, some data reduction is needed together with a two-dimensional presentation. There are two approaches to simplified three-dimensional reconstructions: boundary representation (B-rep) and constructive solid geometry (CSG).

B-rep systems create images by identifying a boundary interface and assembling this as a multiple polyhedral surface: this is rather like fabricating an object by 'tiles' plastered to the surface of a model. The best-known example of this system was developed by Marsh & Vannier (1983) in conjunction with McDonnell-Douglas and implemented on the Siemens CT scanner. CSG systems create an image from a combination of relatively simple solid geometric elements (cubes, polygons etc: the 'Octree' technique). This system has been developed by Phoenix Data Systems (Salyer et al. 1986) on parallel processing equipment. Though the information of the original image is slower by CSG than B-rep, subsequent image manipulation is faster – the functions which have been described as the 'electronic anatomy laboratory'. Simple systems are now also available which run on microcomputer equipment.*

Orthopaedics

Computers, and especially CAD/CAM technology are increasingly used in orthopaedics. Applications include: (1) 3-D reconstructions of skeletal structures; (2) design and simulation of procedures; (3) production of plastic or wax models as templates for preoperative review and sculpting of allografts; and (4) design and manufacture of customised implants (reviewed by Goh et al. 1990 and Pho et al. 1990).†

Stereotactic procedures

Neurosurgery

Sophisticated computer imaging techniques have produced a renaissance in stereotactic surgery. To access a single point in the brain a CT slice is displayed and the target point chosen with a mouse-controlled cursor. Arterial and venous images are then analysed. Finally the optimal surgical trajectory is determined and converted into mechanical adjustments of the stereotactic operating table.

Liver biopsy

An elegant system has been described for construction of a 3-D image of the liver, identifying both vessels and intrahepatic tumours (Hashimoto et al. 1991). This can be used to guide needle puncture for biopsy or treatment.

Surgical applications of virtual reality

Virtual reality is defined as human interaction in an environment simulated by a computer. Possible applications of this have been well reviewed by McGovern (1994). They include simulators for training in minimally invasive surgery, planning of neurosurgical operations, and so-called 'telepresence' surgery in which the surgeon can operate on patients at separate and remote locations.

---

* For example, Orthoplan from Ortho Graphics Inc, 1002 East South Temple, Suite 305, Salt Lake City, UT 84102, USA. This allows the surgeon to manipulate and review a wide variety of orthopaedic procedures on a computer screen.

† The possibilities of complete automation of hip replacement have been elegantly reviewed by Mat Beard in the September 1993 issue of *Personal Computer World* (pp. 499–500).

Diabetic management

The use of computers to monitor blood sugar patterns in diabetic patients has been widely explored. One system enables users to enter data via a special purpose telephone; a voice synthesiser provides immediate feedback including suggestions about adjusting insulin or oral hypoglycaemic therapy (Arbogast & Dodrill 1985). A controlled trial of a simple patient-operated computer system for deciding insulin dosage has been shown to result in lower mean blood glucose values (Peterson et al. 1986). Improved prognosis has been shown in patients monitored by telecommunication and graphical processing of data than in those managed with a traditional diary (Schultz et al. 1992). Delivery of insulin by a programmable pump implanted in the subcutaneous tissue of the abdomen has also been described (Saudek et al. 1989).

Cardiac pacemakers

At one time implantable cardiac pacemakers delivered fixed-rate stimuli to a single chamber. Current devices based on microprocessor technology are far more sophisticated. They can sense and pace both atrial and ventricular electrodes to match a variety of disorders. They can also meet the different functional needs of the patient. For example, the Activitrax pacemaker (Medtronic Inc, Minneapolis, Minn, USA) can automatically increase or decrease heart rate on the basis of activity. An 'intelligent' pacemaker can also store and transmit details of its own performance relative to the underlying cardiac rhythm. The exact requirements can be programmed and the program changed by transmitted instructions.

Psychotherapy

Even though computers are still at a relatively primitive stage of natural language processing, there have been some notable exercises in using them for psychotherapy, beginning with Joseph Weizenbaum's famous ELIZA program in 1966 (Zarr 1984; Erdman et al. 1985).* Most of these systems take advantage of the fact that, in psychiatry, the data collection process itself can be therapeutic: the larger and more detailed the process, the greater the effect. A controlled trial has shown that computer-based behavioural therapy achieves results similar to those of a human therapist. The computer can also be used to encourage patients to talk about their problems, a process which has been referred to as 'computer-assisted soliloquy' (Slack et al. 1990). 'Self-help' programs of this type can provide assistance to individual patients which would not otherwise be available because of cost constraints.

---

* Having been a pioneer of these systems, Weizenbaum now believes that ELIZA may actually be dangerous to users.

The use of an on-line database in treatment

Computer-assisted access to a database is increasingly used in situations involving individual patients (Lindberg et al. 1993). A notable published example was that of a 52-year-old woman undergoing laparotomy for an abdominal mass. Frozen section biopsy revealed this to be 'sclerosing mesenteritis'. Within two minutes a MEDLINE search had provided an up-to-date review on the management of this obscure condition (Sohn & Robbins 1985). This type of procedure will be greatly enhanced by systems for direct interfacing between patient data and MEDLINE (Cimino et al. 1992; Miller et al. 1992).

Nursing

The principles of the use of computers in nursing do not differ in any significant way from those described throughout this book as part of the total clinical process. Indeed, because of the numbers of personnel involved, the majority of clinical computing is likely to be performed by nurses.* There are, however, a small number of specific nursing functions (Table 6.3). Of these, the preparation of a care plan is the most familiar. A care plan should represent a combination of data collection and decision support; some detailed aspects of the computerisation of this process have been reviewed by Evans (1987) and specific software is available (e.g. Nurse Plan Nursing Systems, 76841 Hooton's Corner, Cottage Grove, Oregon 97424, USA).

Table 6.3. Specific nursing functions for which computer-assistance is available

Care plans
Entry and communication of physician orders
Physiological monitoring

Audit

Healthcare providers are under increasing pressure from purchasers (public and private), patients and regulatory agencies to document the quality of the healthcare services provided. Quality-of-care studies (audit) can focus on the structure, the process or the outcome of care. The commonest target is process, comparing the actual care given with that which would have been expected from pre-established criteria. All audit studies should be planned as an 'audit cycle' with the following steps: (1)

---

* An excellent review of this topic is *Nursing Informatics* (eds M. J. Ball, K. J. Hannah, U. G. Jelger and H. Petersen) (1988), Springer-Verlag.

identify standards and performance targets; (2) collect data on current practice; (3) evaluate data relative to standards; and (4) modify practice accordingly. Finally, to 'close the loop' the process should be repeated to ensure that recommendations for change have been implemented. It should be emphasised that a process audit must always involve a comparison. Some current procedures are 'pseudo-audits', merely giving a description of a current system without any element of comparison.

Retrospective enquiries into process from paper-based records demand cumbersome and expensive manual audit. These studies are obviously far faster and more accurate with computer-based records, as demonstrated in an audit of the management of hypertension by General Practitioners in The Netherlands (van der Lei et al. 1991). Indeed, it can reasonably be claimed that the present rapid growth of clinical audit is a direct result of the introduction of computerised systems (Paterson et al. 1991). There is clearly documented evidence that feedback of statistical information can influence clinical practice (Mugford et al. 1991) and an excellent study shows that computer systems can greatly enhance quality assurance in a dialysis program (Pollak 1990). Furthermore, the computerised record also allows for prospective or concurrent audit by incorporation of various prompts and action suggestions to ensure compliance with recommended practice.

7

Computers in medical education

Computers can teach just as well as books but have the added capability of being able to interact with the learner. Computer teaching supplements, but does not replace, the human equivalent. Some aspects of medical research have been revolutionised by computers – especially literature searches.

Introduction

Education can be defined as 'active' when it is delivered by a human teacher to a single student or small group, or 'passive' when it is delivered by 'inanimate' media, such as a book, a television set or a teacher presenting a formal lecture to a large group of students. The key to the use of computers in education is that they go some way towards converting passive into active systems. They do this by providing a degree of quasi-intelligent interaction between the pupil and the medium. The computer can, in effect, conduct a dialogue with the student, leading him through material in a manner which emphasises the relationship among facts as well as the facts themselves, and at a rate which is established by feedback to be the optimum for that individual. A major problem of medical education at present, especially in the preclinical curriculum, is the emphasis on passive systems (i.e. lectures) as against active systems (i.e. tutorial groups) (Michael & Rovick 1986), and computers are expected to contribute towards the solution of this problem.

Interaction is the key new contribution which a computer can bring to education.* There are two further contributions which are less revolutionary but no less important. The first is the ability of the computer to hold vast amounts of rapidly indexed information. This can be structured in a manner which is not easily achieved with traditional media such as books. The machine can move far more rapidly (and therefore effectively) between various aspects of a subject: for example, a surgeon is able to look up an operative procedure together with the relevant anatomy, physiology and medical aspects of the topic. The second major contri-

---

* It is useful to remember the Chinese proverb 'I hear and I forget, I see and I remember, I do and I understand'.

bution is the ability of the computer to provide a simulation of a physiological or pathological situation, and then to modify the model according to the action taken by the student.

Computer-assisted learning (CAL)

This subject is now commonly referred to as computer-assisted learning (CAL) in Europe or computer assisted instruction (CAI) in the US. The general types of computer programs used in medical education are shown in Table 7.1, and examples of specific systems are shown in Table 7.2. At the strictly learning level the two major roles of the computer can be described as those of tutor and laboratory. In the former there is effectively a one-way flow of information to the student; in the latter the computer behaves like a laboratory in which the student can explore different strategies and the results of those strategies. In addition, computers contribute to a variety of educational management functions such as examinations, timetabling, and preparation of audiovisual material. The classification proposed by Cobb (1986) (Table 7.1) will be used for further discussion here.

Table 7.1. Two systems of classification of computer programs used in medical education. In reality, there is often considerable overlap between the different types, and many programs are hybrids

Cobb 1986	Clayden & Wilson 1988
Drill-and-practice	Instructional
Tutorial	Revelatory
Problem-solving	Conjectural
Simulations	Emancipatory
Games	

Drill-and-practice programs

Drill-and-practice programs follow a simple didactic format of presenting a question on a video screen, inviting a response (which may be a true/false, or a multiple choice, or filling in a blank), judging the response and providing some sort of commentary.

Drill-and-practice programs are a very efficient and cost-effective way in which to exercise or develop skills that require straightforward memory. They provide immediate feedback on the answer. The machine can store a great variety of drills and can repeat them endlessly until the material has been mastered. Boredom in the pupil can be avoided by careful design, making use of increasing levels of difficulty, computer-

Table 7.2. Examples of published CAL systems. A detailed review has been published by Cook & McCorkel (1987), and of some of the earlier systems by Piemme (1988)

Topic	Reference
Computer-aided simulation of the clinical environment (CASE) and technological innovations in medical education (TIME)	Harless et al. (1985)
Model of human respiration (MAC series)[a]	Dickinson (1977)
Model of drug metabolism (MACDOPE)[a]	Bloch et al. (1980)
Cardiovascular teaching system (Heartsim)	Rovick & Brenner (1983)
Physiology of muscle	Rovick & Michael (1985); Meiss (1987)
Comprehensive model of human physiology (HUMAN)	Coleman & Randal (1983)
General pathology	Harkin et al. (1986)
Simulation of inhalation anaesthesia (Gas Man)	Philip (1986)
Life support in combat trauma	Henderson et al. (1986)
Biostatistics[b]	
Hypertension[c]	
Graphic presentation of anatomy[d]	Meals & Kabo (1986); Chapman et al. (1992)
Arthritis	Mitchell et al. (1993)

Note that, as with many computer applications, there is a strong tendency to label programs with easily remembered acronyms. This is convenient for users but can become confusing when the total number of published systems is very large. In addition to the formally published CAL systems there are numerous commercial systems covering all areas of preclinical and clinical medicine. This is a difficult area to review because many of these systems, both in the public and the private sector, prove to be ephemeral in either a hardware, software or financial sense.
[a] The MAC series of programs (MacMan [cardiovascular system]; MacPee [renal physiology]; MacPuff [respiration]; MacDope [drug metabolism]) are available from IRL Press at Oxford University Press, Walton Street, Oxford OX2 6DP, UK or Oxford University Press, 200 Madison Avenue, New York, NY 10016, USA.
[b] Available from Elsevier Science Publishing Company Inc, PO Box 1663, Grand Central Station, New York 10163–1663, USA.
[c] Available as part of the CYBERLOG series from Cardinal Health Systems Inc. 7562 Market Place Drive, Eden Prairie, Minnesota 55344–3636, USA.
[d] A simple neuroanatomy project is available from Scholastech Ltd, Britannia House, 1–11 Glenthorne Road, London W6 0LF, UK.

generated animation, sound, colour graphics, and random variation in the drills.

Tutorial programs

Tutorial programs impart new skills and knowledge by a computer-controlled, step-by-step presentation of small pieces of information. At various intervals the presentation is interrupted by a short set of questions to evaluate understanding and to correct any misconceptions. The sequence of material is usually a combination of linear and branching: the program checks the student at certain points; if the response is satisfactory the program moves on to the next section; if the response is not satisfactory the program may return to the beginning of the sequence, or branch to another sequence that gives supplementary material in the area of difficulty.

Problem-solving programs

Programs of the problem-solving type attempt to go further than tutorials by teaching the student how to gather facts and figures, how to evaluate information, and how to formulate logical and appropriate decisions based on that information. This is a type of approach widely adopted in medical education in the form of the clinical case study. A few opening facts are presented ('This is a 28-year-old man with persistent left-sided headache') and the student is asked to choose further questions or investigations. A sophisticated program of this type will allow for a number of different pathways through the information base, rather than slavishly following a single approach. Conceptually this is not unlike the use of production rule systems and cognitive models for computerised medical diagnosis (see Chapter 5); indeed, expert systems such as INTERNIST-1/QMR (Parker & Miller 1989) and Iliad (Turner et al. 1992) have been used as the basis for educational materials. In this way the student can move freely between items of history and items of examination because that more closely mimics the real-life process. The correct conclusion and action are more important than the precise route by which they are achieved.

An excellent example of problem-solving programs is Advanced Clinical Problems on Disk, a joint venture of the American College of Physicians and the Laboratory of Computer Science at the Massachussetts General Hospital (published by William & Wilkins, 428 East Preston Street, Baltimore, MD 21202, USA). This service provides two problems per disk and subscribers receive a new disk every three months.

Simulation programs

Simulation programs provide reinforcement and assessment of performance skills through a model of a real-life situation. The programs may vary from simple mathematical models to elaborate animated audiovisual productions (the flight simulator available as a game on PCs is a good example). In some medical schools simulations are replacing the teaching laboratory in the basic sciences (Meiss 1987; Stephens & Doherty 1992). The traditional approach is expensive in terms of equipment, materials and staff time, and has a doubtful educational return. There are also ethical problems in the use of animals as teaching models. Available simulations include the well-known MAC series of programs (Table 7.2) which provide dynamic models of physiological and pharmacological systems in which related variables can be altered, and the effects calculated and displayed in graphic and text form for further analysis by the student. Simulations are invaluable in allowing real-time simulations of medical and surgical emergencies with a clock running and time as a crucial factor. The combination of microcomputer and videodisk can provide an extraordinary level of realism, with dramatic portrayals of a patient's medical and social conditions (e.g. the TIME system; Harless et al. 1985).

Simulations are among the most valuable of medical teaching aids, in particular because they provide immediate feedback on errors. However, they are always costly and complex to produce. An excellent set of guidelines has been published by Dooling (1987) (Table 7.3).

Educational games

Educational games are a variant on problem-solving programs in which an element of competition is introduced either between the student and the computer, or between students or groups of students. This approach

Table 7.3. The steps involved in designing a computer simulation for education purposes (from Dooling 1987)

Choosing the situation
Defining objectives
Mapping the simulation

Writing the simulation
  Creating the opening scene
  Writing the sections
  Writing the decisions
  Responses/consequences

Scoring

has not been widely used in medical education, perhaps because it might be considered frivolous. Nevertheless, it has been shown to be a very powerful teaching tool in other subjects.

The benefits of CAL

The advantages of CAL are as follows:

1. The computer provides continuous feedback by assessing the student's response and correcting or confirming the answer, branching to other material if necessary. This is the key difference and advantage of CAL over books and audiovisual material.
2. Each individual student can work at his own pace. This solves the familiar problem of group teaching in which the most able students are held back while the least able may never catch up.
3. The computer never tires, has endless patience, and, in principle, is always available. No supervision is necessary.
4. Unlike the instruction given by individual teachers, the quality of instruction given by the computer does not vary. The material is determined by the initial designer or designers and can be subject to the most rigorous process of review and refinement.
5. Unlike books, audiovisual material, and even human teachers, CAL material can be altered and updated quickly and easily. This applies to text material but rather less so to graphics where there may be substantial investment in the original design.
6. High quality teaching material can be readily available on a wide variety of sites, either by postal distribution of disks, or direct connection to a database over telephone lines.
7. Computers can be used for interactive instruction in unusual emergency situations (e.g. life support in combat trauma; Henderson et al. 1986).
8. The use of a CAL system not only instructs in the subject by question but also provides some familiarity with the use of computers in general.

It should be noted that the above advantages apply to a well-designed CAL system. As in all fields of human endeavour, the reality may fall short of the ideal. For example, the advantages of availability to the individual may have little meaning if there is only one terminal which is accessible only during office hours.

The acceptability of CAL systems

Almost every study which has addressed student attitudes to CAL has yielded favourable results (reviewed by Prentice & Kenny 1986). However, 'favourable' means that a majority of students gave a positive response, which still leaves a minority who consider that the computer is a poor teaching medium or at least difficult to use. Furthermore, it is difficult to assess 'attitudes' to CAL in a useful and realistic manner, even though there have been some notable efforts to do so (Xakellis & Gjerde 1990). It must be accepted that CAL will probably happen regardless of whether it is supported by a large or a small majority.

The efficacy of CAL systems

As with attitudes, it is difficult to make a completely objective assessment of the efficacy of a CAL system. Most studies which have attempted some sort of controlled comparison have concluded that CAL is equal or superior to other systems (reviewed by Prentice & Kenny 1986). Examples include a reduction in the time taken to learn gross anatomy (Marion et al. 1982), and improvement in test scores in pharmacology (Pazdernik & Walaszek 1983). The feedback capabilities of the computer are particularly important in this respect (Wigton et al. 1986). However, the difficulty with many studies of this type is that they may be biassed by the inevitable enthusiasm of the investigator who is usually also the designer of the system under test. Some critics are less enthusiastic. A comparison of anatomy teaching by interactive videodisc with that of traditional cadaver demonstration showed no difference in student performance (Guy & Frisby 1992). Others have found CAL to be less effective than a traditional tutorial (Garrett et al. 1987). In addition there is often a problem with portability, i.e. the system works well in the hands of the originator, but is difficult to implement on other sites.

Factors restraining the implementation of CAL systems

Given the clearcut advantages of CAL, what are the obstacles to its immediate implementation in all medical schools? These are cost, resistance by educators or students, and availability. Cost may have been an obstacle to the prototype mainframe-based systems of the 1970s but plays no significant part in the 1990s. There is no reason why every medical student should not have their own microcomputer for both stand-alone operation or connection as a terminal. The price would be a small fraction of the extremely high costs of medical education. Resistance by staff or students is also a minor, probably non-existent factor. Today it requires little effort to 'sell' the concept of computing in any field. Questions of reliability and ease of use have also been substantially answered in the current generation of hardware and software. The major problem of implementation is undoubtedly that of availability of authoritative, cost-effective material which will run on a wide variety of equipment. Coupled with this is the problem of knowing what is available, since there are no standard catalogues such as those which exist for books and journals.

Programs for conducting tests

Computers can be used to automate the whole process of setting and scoring a test. The programs consist of a large database of test items and a means for the random selection of a subset of items. They may also include means for checking the answers and evaluating the final score.*

In terms of computerisation the simplest and most widely exploited question is the multiple-choice type, where the response entry is a single character (e.g. 't' for true, 'f' for false, or a number from a list). Rather more complex, but essential to a flexible system, is the ability of a program to accept complete words or parts of words as responses. It is more complex because most medical terms have synonyms: for example, if the answer to a question is 'Crohn's disease' the computer must also accept 'regional ileitis'. Because students are not necessarily typists, it is common to make use of the shortest word root which would be unambiguous (e.g. 'Cro' or 'reg'). Similarly, some questions may request a numerical answer, the response being accepted if it lies within a predetermined range of normal values.

Computers are now quite widely used for setting and scoring examinations. However, the actual test itself is still almost always a paper exercise, often a box-and-tick questionnaire which can be assessed by an optical character reader (OCR) connected to a computer. The use of interactive terminals for testing will undoubtedly become more common. In the US, the National Board of Examiners has developed a computer-based examination called CBX which presents a complex patient simulation requiring diagnosis and management. The efficiency of systems of this type has been examined: approximately nine cases are needed to achieve an adequate level of reliability in measuring the problem-solving ability of a student or resident (Diserens et al. 1986), and the final results correlate well with other measures (Clyman et al. 1992).

An interesting development is that of 'adaptive' testing. If a question is answered correctly a more difficult question is asked; if the answer is incorrect a simple question is presented. In effect, the computer can dwell on an area until it is certain whether or not the candidate's performance falls above or below the pass-fail line (Melnick 1986).

Word processing and graphics

Though not strictly 'educational', word-processing makes a major practical contribution to the production of class handouts, examinations, reports and timetables. Simple though it may appear, this is probably the major present function of the computer in educational systems.

---

* The range of shell testing programs by QuestionMark Computing (12 Heath Villas, London NW3 1AW, UK) is particularly commended.

Equally important is the rapidly growing field of graphics preparation for teaching purposes. Machines such as the Apple Macintosh can reduce by 25–75 per cent the labour required to produce text slides and charts, as can PC programs such as Harvard Graphics (SPC Software Publishing, 1901 Landings Drive, PO Box 7210, Mountain View, CA 94039, USA). A wide variety of ready-made anatomical and medical images are also available on disk (e.g. Mediclip from Mosby, 11830 Westline Industrial Drive, St. Louis, MO 63146, USA). Preparation of teaching material is one of the best current practical uses of the so-called desk top-publishing (DTP) systems. However, the use of a DTP program is sometimes less easy than the advertisements might suggest. Laidlaw (1989) has set out a series of practical rules for beginners in this area. Chao & Chao (1990) have published a useful review of currently available packages.

Hypertext

There has been a minor revolution in CAL with the increasing use of Hypertext. This is not the easiest of concepts to grasp without hands-on experience: once tried, however, its value seems blindingly obvious. The general definition of Hypertext is that it is a system which allows the user to create links between items of information in a text and to navigate through different texts using these links. Links can be made between words, phrases or even paragraphs. When the links extend to graphics, the term Hypermedia is used. By way of example, picture a screen of text describing side-effects of antibiotics. This text includes the word 'allergy'. The word is selected (typically, by pointing with a mouse) whereupon a list appears of all other screens containing the word 'allergy'. These may include definitions, causes, pathology, etc. Assume that pathology is selected and that this screen includes the words 'mast cell': clicking on this then introduces further screens with references to mast cells. In this way the student can browse through large volumes of information in a self-directed and highly convenient manner.

The best known Hypertext package is Hypercard, available on the Apple Macintosh series. The existence of this package goes a long way to explaining the great appeal of Apple machines in teaching institutions. Other similar programs are available for PC equipment, notably GUIDE (Office Work-stations Ltd, Rosebank House, 144 Broughton Road, Edinburgh EH7 4LE, UK).

Excellent reviews of the use of Hypertext have been provided by Hardman (1990) and Frisse (1990).

Authoring programs

Authoring programs are 'shell' programs which permit the educator with little or no computer experience to create new educational material

Table 7.4. Examples of published authoring programs which provide a 'shell' for the development of CAL systems

Program	Reference
Programmed inquiry learning or teaching (PILOT) – a dialect of Pascal	Richards (1984)
Preparation of a sequence of test screens (MACGEN)	Utsch & Ingram (1978)
TUTOR language which provided material for the PLATO system	Levy 1989

(Baker 1987). Many of the earlier systems were designed to overcome the educational disadvantages of using centralised, batch-processing mainframe computers. In an age of interactive terminals and microcomputers this is now irrelevant. Indeed, given the current availability of simple and flexible high-level languages, some have even questioned whether there is any need at all for specific authoring programs.

A good example of an authoring program is MACGEN (Utsch & Ingram 1978) in which programs are constructed as a sequence of screens. The author enters text, questions or scores as appropriate. Other examples of authoring programs are shown in Table 7.4. Excellent accounts of the detailed steps involved in producing CAL programs and simulations have been published by Joseph & Joseph (1985) and Dooling (1987).

Equipment required for CAL systems

In general the equipment required for CAL systems does not differ from that in other areas of medical computing. However, there are certain differences of emphasis:

1. *Learning* is often performed by an individual working on his or her own and is therefore particularly well suited to a microcomputer.
2. *Memory requirement* is static rather than dynamic, i.e. large amounts of information may be called upon but little if any input is required. The floppy disk has proved a useful medium for education because of its portability. Increasing use is being made of high-density media such as laser-read disks. The 12 inch videodisc (Philips Laservision) can store 54 000 frames per side, each equivalent to a 35 mm slide image. Played at 30 frames per second, each slide can provide 30 minutes of motion picture. Any single frame can be random-accessed in less than 3 seconds. A segment of instruction can be presented by the computer, with a video and audio feedback, in around 1 second. The CD-ROM plays a similar role. Unlike Laservision the information is transferred in digital rather than analog mode, and the speed is therefore not sufficient to support full animation. However, it is ideal for textual information. The standard 4.72 inch CD-ROM can hold up to 550

megabytes of digitally stored information – roughly equivalent to the entire text of the library of 190 books recommended to the internist by the American College of Physicians.

3. *Computational speed* is usually unimportant (though the rate of search through databases may be).

4. *Graphics.* Sophisticated graphics and audiovisual effects are (or should be) a key part of CAL systems. This is in contrast to most other medical systems where simple text and numbers are usually sufficient. The need for graphics is another strong argument for the use of micro-computers where these facilities are much more powerful and readily available than with terminals to larger systems.

5. *Video presentation.* Combinations of computers and video material are highly desirable. Computer-controlled random-access slide projectors or videotape have been used for this purpose but tend to be slow. The videodisc is much superior to videotape in terms of quality and speed. However, the expense of producing discs is high (at least $10 000 (£6000)) and mass production is essential to keep costs to a reasonable level. This requires a degree of consensus on the content of the teaching material which is unusual in medical education. Most current clinical videodisc material has been sponsored by pharmaceutical companies for quasi-promotional purposes (Culbert et al. 1989).

A valuable account of the design and implementation of a computer learning centre in a medical school has been published by Lloyd et al. (1989).

Distance learning: teleconferencing

The concept of linking several people on several sites with a 'conference call' is already very familiar. Current technology is now extending this to video images so that the teacher can communicate, in real-time, with an audience which may be separated by thousands of miles. This is expensive (c. $3000 (£2000) per hour), but like most other advanced communication modalities the price will fall and give much more scope for its use in education. The possibility of using computer networks, such as JANET in the UK and INTERNET in the US for long-distance discussion groups is now being explored in a wide variety of clinical topics (reviewed by Parsons 1989).

Computers and educational philosophy

The introduction of a new educational technique will always lead to a re-opening of old arguments about educational philosophy. In the field of CAL this argument rotates around the two extreme approaches to skill acquisition put forward by Papert on the one hand and Gallwey on the other. Seymour Papert advocates a learning environment in which the learner is constantly faced with new problems and the need to discover new rules. To this end, Papert devised a computer language known as Logo the main purpose of which was to teach 'procedural thinking' to small children. Gallwey, by contrast, aims for an environment in which there are no such problems and therefore no need for analytic reflection.

The value of Papert's model is that problems may arise at any stage of learning which require rational analytic thought. Gallwey's insight is that skill in any domain is measured by the ability to act appropriately in situations that are no longer problems and thus do not require analytic reflection. The Gallwey approach might leave the expert without the means to solve new problems but the Papert approach could leave the learner as a perpetual beginner dependent on rules and analysis, thus blocking the acquisition of expertise.

Another area of quasi-philosophical discussion concerns the supposed deficiencies of books as educational tools. Most medical books are organised by diseases and the clinical findings appear as subheadings under individual conditions. By contrast, real life clinical problems present themselves in the reverse order, i.e. as a set of findings from which a disease must be elucidated. Some books of differential diagnosis are available, but usually deal with only one or two findings at a time, not large combinations. A computer 'textbook' provides the opportunity to create an information network where related pieces of information can be examined in complex arrays from a number of different viewpoints. This criticism of books, however, ignores the fact that the mind of the trained physician constitutes its own network perfectly capable of organising information regardless of the aspect presented.

The present and future place of computers in medical education

The total amount of CAL in current use in medical education is very small. Nevertheless, despite some critical voices (Golden & Friedlander 1987), it is difficult to conceive a future in which computers do not play an important role in medical teaching. They are, for example, an integral part of the new 'caring' curriculum which is being introduced at Harvard Medical School. At the same time the role of computers should not be over-estimated. They are not a panacea for all other problems but should rather be regarded as an adjunct to human instruction which will, in the fullness of time, have a function and importance similar to that of printed books.

Computers in patient education

Computers can be used to educate patients as well as professionals. Examples include instruction in the collection of an uncontaminated midstream urine specimen (Fisher et al. 1977), a system designed to ensure better patient compliance in the use of tricyclic antidepressants

(Sorrell et al. 1982) and a system to educate asthma patients which has been shown to reduce morbidity and hospital admissions (Osman et al. 1994). In the Cleveland area of the US a computerised bulletin board has been set up so that anyone with access to a terminal and modem can send messages and questions. Physicians monitor the system and answer whatever questions come in. This scheme has revealed a substantial demand for an anonymous information source of this type. Health-related programs are also available from the large general information utilities, such as CARE (on The Source) and Health-Tex (on CompuServe). A very useful Index of Health Education Micro-computer Programs is available from the Computer Centre (The Queen's College, 1 Park Drive, Glasgow C3 6LP, UK).

Teaching computing to medical students

With the great increase in the use of computers in all branches of medicine it is logical to include computing as an item in the curriculum of all health-care professionals. Courses in interactive computing have been described for medical students (Hasman 1982; Skiba 1985) and a detailed set of objectives has been proposed by Jelovsek (1988). The rapid growth in the use of microcomputers by medical students has been documented by Haynes and colleagues (1993). It is important to recognise that computer literacy among medical professionals should focus on what computers do (i.e. medical informatics) rather than how they do it. There is certainly no need for the non-specialist to learn any programming language in detail. The strongest case for computer literacy is the 'problem solving process related to information processing that has been spawned by computers' (Evans 1985). Evans has proposed that the three areas which should be addressed in teaching computing to health professionals are database-development and management, expert system development, and simulations.

Teaching computing to physicians

The guidelines for teaching qualified physicians are virtually the same as those for medical students. In addition, there are packages which provide specific and practical help for the physician who wishes to computerise his practice (e.g. Medical Practice Automation Videotape from Master Computer Video Inc, 600 South Cherry Street, Denver, CO 80222, USA). Appeals are being made for the establishment of academic departments of medical informatics in every teaching institution (Greenes & Shortliffe 1990).

Training staff in computer use

This is one of the most essential features of the installation of a new computer system, yet its importance is frequently overlooked. In a large institution the 'cascade' method is usually adopted. Key senior personnel are trained by expert computer staff. These key trainers are then themselves responsible for the instruction of a team of more junior staff.

Some institutions now run specific courses in medical computing: for example, the MSc course offered by the University of Wales (Department of Medical Computing & Statistics, University of Wales College of Medicine, Heath Park, Cardiff CF4 4XN); City University (Department of Systems Science, Northampton Square, London EC1V 0HB); and the University of Warwick (Health Information Science Courses, School of Postgraduate Medical Education, Coventry CV4 7AL).

Medical dictionaries

The classical medical dictionary is an obvious target for conversion to electronic format. *Stedman's Medical Dictionary* is now available on a floppy disk (Williams & Wilkins Electronic Media, 428 Preston Street, Baltimore, MD 21202, USA).

On-line medical information services

With the rapid advances in communications technology, increasing use is being made of central databases for education, research and routine clinical practice (Wyatt 1991). Several thousand such databases are available, and some of the better known are listed in Table 7.5.

Computerised databases are not merely a convenient way of searching for information. They are rapidly becoming essential given that the amount of scientific information is increasing by 13 per cent per year and the total database is doubling every 5.5 years. Nearly half of all users of MEDLINE are now individuals rather than institutions (Wallingford et al. 1990).

For the small investment in a modem, any microcomputer with an RS-232 serial port can be linked via the public telephone network to these databases and this has been described as 'perhaps the most successful application of computers in medicine' (Wyatt 1991). The services can be described under three headings: MEDLARS (MEDLINE), and its European-based competitor *Excerpta Medica*; commercial databases; and institutional databases. However, there is very considerable overlap among these: in particular, most of the commercial suppliers act as a 'gateway' to the products of all the other groups.

MEDLARS (MEDLINE)

MEDLARS (MEDLINE) is the best known of the medical databases and has been described as 'perhaps the most successful application of computers in medicine'. (Wyatt 1991). It was started by the National Library of

Medicine (NLM) in Washington in the 1960s, with the aim of developing a computer system for publishing *Index Medicus*; this was the Medical Literature Analysis and Retrieval System (MEDLARS). Subsequently, this database was made available for on-line enquiries (MEDLINE) (reviewed by Bickers 1985a, b). The files date back to 1966 and include some 6 million articles from over 3500 journals. Abstracts have been available since 1975. Systems for direct interfacing between individual patient data and a MEDLINE search are under intense development (Cimino et al. 1993).

Excerpta Medica

The European-based bibliographic database *Excerpta Medica* is the single major competitor to MEDLINE, from which it differs by the inclusion of some professionally written abstracts and a different profile of journals referenced. It is available through DIALOG and BRS (see below) (Table 7.5).

Commercial database services

There are a variety of commercial database suppliers, who usually include MEDLINE and *Excerpta Medica* amongst their offerings. The relative advantages and disadvantages of these have been reviewed by Bickers (1985b). One of the most obvious variables is the cost of connection time (ranging from $0.40 to $5.00 (25 pence to £3.25) per minute), but other variables, such as search speeds and modem speeds, and the ease of search, renders any simple comparison meaningless.

Broadly speaking, any one of the major suppliers such as DIALOG or BRS should give the average physician access to all the information they are likely to need.

DIALOG

DIALOG Information Services (Lockheed Corporation) is the World's largest supplier of general on-line database information (Table 7.5). The MEDLINE files constitute about 4 per cent of the total and other medical and bioscience files constitute 9 per cent. The access system Knowledge Index has been particularly commended for its efficiency and simplicity.

Bibliographic Retrieval Services (BRS)

BRS is very similar to DIALOG, but makes something of a speciality of medicine and the biosciences. Unlike MEDLINE, BRS offers files which link several databases – for example, medicine and economics – and a SuperIndex which is a compilation of the index pages from nearly 2000 leading reference books. Furthermore, BRS also offers the complete text

Table 7.5. Names, addresses and telephone numbers of some on-line databases
which provide medical material

AMA/GTE Telenet Medical Information Network
8229 Boone Boulevard, Vienna VA 22180, USA

Bibliographic Retrieval Services (BRS)
(including BRS After Dark and BRS Colleague (Medical))
1200 Route 7, Latham, NY 12110, USA
800–553–5566 or 800–833–4707

CompuServe Information Service
5000 Arlington Centre Boulevard, Columbus, OH 43220, USA

DIALOG Information Services Inc.
Marketing Department, 3460 Hillview Avenue, Palo Alto, CA 94304, USA
800–227–5510

MEDLARS (MEDLINE) Management Section,
National Library of Medicine, 8600 Rockville Pike
Bethesda, MD 20209
301–496–6193

The Source Telecomputing Corporation,
1616 Anderson Road, McLean VA 22101, USA

International Pharmaceutical Abstracts,
American Society of Hospital Pharmacists,
4630 Montgomery Avenue, Bethesda, MD 20814, USA

PDQ Information Coordinator,
International Cancer Information Center, Office of
International Affairs, National Cancer Institute,
Building 82, Room 103, Bethesda, MD 20894, USA
301–496–7403

Fondation Suisse TELMED,
Rue Pedro-Meylan 7, Case Postale 260, 1211 Geneva 17, Switzerland

DERM/INFONET
Dermatology Services Inc.
American Academy of Dermatology, 1567 Maple Avenue,
Evanston, IL 60201, USA
321–869–3954

MEDIS
MeadDataGeneral, 9393 Springboro Pike, PO Box 933, Dayton, OH 45401, USA
800–227–4908

Paper Chase
Beth Israel Hospital, 330 Brookline Avenue, Boston, MA 02215, USA
617–735–2253

Combined Health Information Database (CHID) (health education materials)
Herner & Company, 1700 North Moore Street, Arlington, VA 22209, USA

Current Contents on Diskette
Institute for Scientific Information
132 High Street, Uxbridge, Middlesex UB8 1DP, UK
+44 895 70016

Table 7.5. continued

World Research Database
Longman/Microinfo Ltd, PO Box 3, Omega Park, Alton, Hampshire GU 34 2PG,
UK
0420 86848

Connection to these databases requires a computer, a modem and an account number and password; the latter are obtained by writing directly to the service. Many are also now available on CD-ROM. A current list of databases in the US is available from Information USA Computer Data Service, 12400 Bell Mountain Road, Potomac, MD 20854, USA. A very detailed list also appears in Dalton (1990).

of many journal articles and medical textbooks (The BRS Colleague system) (Table 7.5).

Institutional database services

Institutional database services are very similar to the commercial services in overall scope and use, but add an element of organisational 'quality control'.

AMA/GTE Telenet Medical Information Network (MINET)

The major content of MINET is American Medical Association publications in a constantly updated database format. The 'Drug Evaluations' database is very highly regarded.

Paper Chase

Paper Chase was developed at Beth Israel hospital in Boston, and provides on-line searches of that hospital's library holdings (Underhill & Bleich 1986) (Table 7.5). The success is due to the 'intelligence' and friendliness of the user interface which permits users to enter search terms without regard for standardised subject headings or abbreviations.

Medical Special Interest Group (MedSIG)

MedSIG is a group of miscellaneous features, including medical programs and bulletin boards available through general purpose services such as CompuServe and The Source and sponsored by the American Association for Medical Systems and Informatics (AAMSI). Many local areas in the US also operate medical bulletin boards.

Patient Data Query (PDQ) system

PDQ is a clinically oriented database provided by the National Cancer Institute that makes available state-of-the-art information on cancer treatment which is updated monthly by an editorial board (Table 7.5). It also includes a file of cancer-research protocols (controlled trials) and a directory of physicians and organisations providing cancer care (Hubbard et al. 1987).

DERM/INFONET

This is a group of databases of special dermatological interest, including a subset of MEDLINE and various management aids (Table 7.5).

ADONIS

The ADONIS CD-ROM Biomedical collection is a full-text collection of over 200 biomedical journals. Laser-printed copies of this literature are available from the British Library, Document Centre in the UK and Information on Demand Inc in the USA (Information on Demand Inc, PO Box 1370, Berkeley, CA 94701, USA; tel. 1–800/227–0750).

CDC Wonder

An on-line public health information service from the Centers for Disease Control and Prevention (Friede et al. 1993).

Which database?

The choice of database or access route can be very confusing. As a broad generalisation, there is a direct relationship between cost and speed, and an inverse relationship between both of these and ease of use. In one comparative study (Haynes et al. 1985) a search was made of the MEDLINE databases for information on prescribing Timolol after myocardial infarction. The costs were \$3.38 for NLM, \$6.58 for COLLEAGUE and \$11.62 for Paper Chase; the times were 6.26, 12.11 and 18.32 minutes respectively; and difficulty of use (on a scale of 0 to 7 with 7 being the hardest) was rated at 3.7, 2.7 and 1.0 respectively. Because of the costs and complexity there have been some rather negative reports on the use of on-line databases by individual clinicians. However, technical advances are rapidly solving most of these problems (except costs).

Bulletin boards

A bulletin board is a computer system set up to allow multiple users access to data via telephone lines. Facilities typically include electronic mail and conferencing. This rapidly advancing topic has been reviewed by Spencer & Sampson (1992).

Reference retrieval

One of the most valuable pieces of software in academic medicine is a reference manager (Jones 1993). These can take in references from a number of sources (manual, CD-ROM etc.) and output them in a format appropriate to different journals (Vancouver system, Harvard system etc.). This author uses the system available from Research Information Systems, 2355 Camino Vida Rable, Carlsbad, CA 92009-1572, USA; tel. 619-438 5526.

8

Miscellaneous applications of computers in medicine and related topics

> The use of computers in medicine has provided a major stimulus to the development of standardised medical terminology

There are a variety of applications of computers in medicine and related fields that cannot readily be classified under the headings of the previous sections. Some of these are summarised in Table 8.1.

Computers in molecular biology

One notable area of research application is molecular biology. A number of databases/networks have been created that serve a variety of functions including the assembly of large scale DNA sequences and a search of the database for similarities with existing sequences.* Suppliers of these systems are listed in Table 8.2. In the US a national database has been prepared to enable tracking of violent criminals by DNA typing profiles (Baechtel et al. 1991).

Modelling of biological and clinical situations

Computer models of clinical situations are widely used for educational purposes but the operation and output of such programs are fixed by the original design. Computer models have also been designed in which the outcome is not known, the whole purpose of the system being to ascertain outcomes in relation to different inputs and assumptions. These models often use the random number generator of the computer in order to implement the so-called Monte Carlo simulation techniques. Examples of such models include abdominal pain (de Dombal et al. 1971), pelvic infections (Chard 1987), and clinical laboratory procedures (Connelly & Willard 1989). In the biological field an especially elegant example is the model of evolution designed by Dawkins (1986) which shows how cumulative selection can generate substantial changes within a relatively few generations of apparently random variation. In the administrative field

---

* An issue of *Nucleic Acids Research* (Vol. 16, No. 5, Part A, 1988) and of *Biotechniques* (Vol. 10, No 6, 1991) are devoted to the application of computers to research on nucleic acids.

142

Table 8.1. Some useful reviews and references to miscellaneous applications
of computers in topics related to medicine

Application	Reference
Calculation of genetic distance and heritability	Sattler & Hilburn (1985) Vandemark et al. (1985) Cowen et al. (1985)
Predicting toxicity and carcinogenicity of chemical compounds	Franke et al. (1985) Klopman (1985)
Dentistry	Stikeleather et al. (1988)[a]
Post-marketing surveillance of adverse drug reactions	Hall et al. (1988)
Computers in medical libraries	Matheson (1986)
Operating room schedules	Ball et al. (1986)
Clinical trials in psychopharmacology	Severe (1987)
Theoretical chemistry ('designer drugs')	McCammon (1988) Howard & Kollman (1988) Martin (1991)
Reproductive toxicology	Scialli (1988)
Nutrient database	Schakel et al. (1988)
Protein engineering	van Gunsteren (1988)
Forensic medicine	Sivaloganathan (1987)
Quantification of scalp hair	Gibbons & Fiedler-Weiss (1986)
Chromatography	Various authors (1989)[b]
Dermatology	Various authors (1989)[c]
Clinical genetics	Winter (1990)
Estimating the time of death	Lynnerup 1993
Parasite identification	Theodoropoules et al. 1993

[a] In an issue of *Dental Clinics in North America* devoted to this topic (Vol. 32, No. 1, January 1988.

[b] 'Computer-assisted method development in chromatography' (*Journal of Chromatography*, Vol. 485, 1989).

[c] 'Computers & Dermatology' (*Seminars in Dermatology*, Vol. 18, No. 2, 1989)

models are used to assess economic scenarios: an interesting example was a computer simulation of the financial impact of smoking by hospital nurses, together with the effect of various programs for reducing smoking (Swank et al. 1988). The use of models in treatment (surgery, radiotherapy) has already been reviewed in Chapter 6.

Standardisation of medical terminology

The increasing use of computer systems in medical administration, data collection and research has added greatly to demands for a single

Table 8.2. Examples of databases/networks which provide material related to nucleic acids research. The Human Genome Project, in particular, is generating vast quantities of data together with disputes as to how it should be handled (Aldhous 1991; Barsalov & Brutlag 1991)

Name	Address
Gen-Bank	RBN Laboratories Inc, 10 Moulton Street, Cambridge, MA 02238, USA
EMBL	European Molecular Biology Laboratory, Meyerhofstrasse 1, 6900 Heidelberg, FRG
GENOFIT	Case Postale 239, 1212 Grand-Lancy, Geneva, Switzerland
DNASTAR	1801 University Avenue, Madison, WI 53705, USA

coherent system of medical terminology. Several systems have been described and the best known of these are listed in Table 8.3. The classification of human disease is an important and major exercise in its own right. Blois (1984) has shown how a disease can be described as a name (N) or by attributes (A)* or by a combination of the two (N ∥ A). For example, a description of influenza might need (influenza ∥ fever, sore-throat, viral infection, ... etc). ICD codes use the name alone (N ∥); the disease names are standardised, linked with synonyms, and given a number. SNOP user attributes alone (∥ A); the attributes are given in standard form and numbered. SNOMED combines both names and attributes (N ∥ A).

The best known classification is the ICD system introduced by the World Health Organization in 1946 (reviewed by Cote & Rothwell 1989). The current edition (ICD-9) was adopted in 1976; ICD-10 is expected in 1994. In the US, further detail is added as the ICD-9-CM. ICD-9 contains 9607 terms and uses up to four character codes; ICD-9-CM has 10 845 terms and allows six digit codes.

Although the ICD system is still the most widely used classification it has the disadvantage of being a single-axis system, dealing only with disease names. Each concept has to be coded with a separate number, leading to overcrowding within four digits and a loss of detail. The major

---

* Each disease will typically have a number of attributes (clinical features) so that A is, in fact, $(A^1, A^2, A^3, ... A^n)$.

† SNOMED. *Coding Manual*; alphabetical index; numerical index. 2nd edn. Skokie, Illinois: College of American Pathologists (1979).

Table 8.3. Systems of medical terminology. Excellent reviews, including history, are Cote & Rothwell (1989) and Bishop (1989)

System	Comments
International Statistical Classification of Diseases, Injury and Causes of Death (ICD)	The most widely used system but single axis (disease names only). See text.
Systematised Nomenclature of Pathology (SNOP)	A multi-axis system developed by the American College of Pathologists, which subsequently evolved into SNOMED.
Systematised Nomenclature of Medicine (SNOMED)	A further development of SNOP, and may become the definitive system of classification.
Medical Subject Heading (MeSH)	Developed by the National Library of Medicine (NLM).
Current Procedural Terminology (CPT-4)	Widely used in the US by private insurers.
Heath Care Procedural Coding System (HCPCS)	Used by Medicare.
Unified Medical Language System	Developed by the NLM as the most advanced system to link all others.
Read Clinical Classification (RCC)	A universal classification system developed in the UK.
The Arden Syntax	A standard of the American Society of Testing and Materials for representing medical knowledge.

alternative is SNOMED which is a multi-axis system classifying a number of aspects of the disease. SNOMED† codes on seven separate axes: topography, morphology, cause, function, disease, procedures and occupation (Cote & Rothwell 1989). The latest version of SNOMED (SNOMED III) will also attempt to integrate all the ICD rubrics and codes at the level of the disease classification axis.

One major problem of classification is that different systems often use different terms for the same condition: examples of differences between MeSH and SNOMED have been documented by Hersh & Greenes (1990). The National Library of Medicine (NLM) has initiated a project to develop a Unified Medical Language (UML) (Humphreys & Lindberg 1993). The goal of this is to develop a 'meta-thesaurus' that will allow translation of terms between different vocabularies. The first version of UML contains 66 000 distinct concepts and 97 700 terms including synonyms and variants.* A similar approach, together with a five level hierarchical system for the description of all aspects of a disease, has been developed by Read in the UK.†

It is generally agreed that the user interface of medical computing systems should be based on natural language and that medical data should then be automatically encoded by the machine (Cote & Rothwell 1989). The highly desirable aim of extracting data from medical texts and translating from one system to another is being pursued by a number of groups (Cimino & Barnett 1990; Hersh & Greenes 1990) but practical examples are still rare.

Some authors have presented models of medical data organisation which centre around the 'medical event' as the most fundamental item. The medical event has three dimensions: a dimension of patients (identification of the individual), a dimension of time (series of events); and a dimension of medical knowledge, where the latter is a data dictionary or vocabulary of all medical terms (clinical features, diagnoses, treatment etc.). Within this concept the aim becomes to define a total and all embracing data dictionary, including all synonyms (Linnarsson & Wigertz 1989).

Standardisation of clinical data transmission

Work on standardisation of terminology is closely paralleled by work on interchange of clinical and laboratory data between computers. Major initiatives in this area are listed in Table 8.4.

---

* UML is available on CD-ROM from Betsy Humphreys, Library Operations, National Library of Medicine, 8600 Rockville Pike, Bethesda, MD 20209, USA.

† Read codes are available from Computer Aided Medical Systems Ltd, 26–28 Leicester Road, Loughborough, Leicestershire LE11 2AG, UK.

Table 8.4. Standards for exchange of medical data between different computer systems

Name	Features
American Society for Testing Materials 1238[a]	Transmission of laboratory data with extension to clinical observations including United Medical Language (UML) and the Arden syntax.
ASTM E-1381 and E-1394	Linking clinical and laboratory instruments to other systems.
Health Level 7 (HL7)[b]	Transmission of admission, discharge, administration and charge information.
Euclides (CEN-001)[c]	European initiative for the standardisation of laboratory data interchange.
CEN Technical Committee 251	European initiative for development of a general set of standards for health care information.

[a] ASTM, 1916 Race Street, Philadelphia, PA 19103, USA.
[b] W E Hammond, Duke University, Box 2914, Durham, NC 27710, USA.
[c] G de Moor, State University Hospital of Ghent, Department of Medical Informatics, De Pintelaan 185, 9000 Ghent, Belgium.

General reading on computers in medicine

Journals

British Journal of Healthcare Computing
BJHC Books, 45 Woodland Grove, Weybridge, Surrey KT13 9EQ, UK.

Computers in Biology & Medicine
Pergamon Journals Ltd, Headington Hill Hall, Oxford OX3 0BW, UK.

Computers in Healthcare
Cardiff Publishing Co., 6430 South Yosemite Street, Englewood, CO 80111, USA.

Computers in Nursing
J B Lippincott Company, 2350 Virginia Avenue, Hagerstown, MD 21740, USA.

Computer Applications in the Biosciences
IRL Press Ltd, PO Box 1, Eynsham, Oxford OX8 1JJ, UK.

MD Computing
Springer-Verlag Service Center Secaucus, 44 Hartz Way, Secaucus, NJ 07094, USA.

Medical Decision Making
Birkhauser Boston Inc, 380 Green Street, Cambridge, MA 02129, USA.

The Journal of International Biomedical Information and Data (IBID),
33 Vale Road, Tunbridge Wells, Kent TN1 1BP, UK.

Methods of Information in Medicine
F. K. Schattauer Verlag GmbH, 7 Stuttgart 1, Postfach 2945, Lenzhalde 3, FRG.

Biomedicial Measurement Informatics & Control
87 Gower Street, London WC1E 6AA, UK.

International Journal of Clinical Monitoring & Computing
PO Box 163, 3300 AD Dordrecht, The Netherlands.

A very detailed list of medical informatics journals appeared in *Biomedica Informatics Today*, Vol. 17, No. 7, 1993.

Books

Benson T (1991) *Medical Informatics*. Longman, Harlow.
Dalton KJ, Chard T (1990) Computers in obstetrics and gynaecology. Elsevier, Amsterdam.
Illingworth D, Glaser EL, Pyle IC (eds) (1986) Dictionary of computing. Oxford University Press, Oxford.
Preece J (1990) The use of computers in general practice. Churchill Livingstone, London.

Reggia JA, Tuhrim S (eds) (1985) Computer assisted decision making (2 vols). Springer-Verlag, New York.
Rowley, D, Purser H (1988) Clinical information technology. Taylor & Francis, London.
Shortcliffe EH, Perreault LE (1990) Medical informatics: computer applications in heath care. Addison-Wesley. Reading, MA.

Other sources of information

A directory on disk of information sources, products and services related to medical computing (*CIBA-Geigy Medical Computing Resource Guide*) is available from Resource Systems Management Ind, 3300 Mitchell Lane, Suite 390, Boulder, CO 80301, USA).

Detailed reviews of individual software packages, either general or medical, have not been attempted here because they are certain to become out-of-date during the lifetime of this book. Journals are the best source of current reviews, especially those which are published on a regular basis in *MD Computing*. (*MD Computing* (1993) The 10th annual directory of medical hardware and software companies **10**, 231–267.)

References

Adams, I. D., Chan, M., Clifford, P. C., Cooke, W. M., Dallos, V., de Dombal, F. T., Edwards, M. H., Hancock, D. M., Hewett, D. J., McIntyre, N., Somerville, P. G., Spiegelhalter, D. J., Welwood, J. and Wilson, D. H. (1986) Computer aided diagnosis of acute abdominal pain: a multicenter study. British Medical Journal **293**, 800–804.

Aldhous, P. (1991) Human genome databases at the crossroads. Nature **352**, 94.

Alemi, F., Cherry, F. and Meffert, G. (1989) Rehearsing decisions may help teenagers: an evaluation of a simulation game. Computers in Biology and Medicine **19**, 283–290.

Alvey, P. L., Myers, C. D. and Greaves, M. F. (1987a) High performance for expert systems: I. Escaping from the demonstrator class. Medical Informatics **12**, 85–95.

Alvey, P. L., Presont, N. J. and Greaves, M. F. (1987b) High performance for expert systems: II. A system for leukaemia diagnosis. Medical Informatics **12**, 97–114.

American Psychiatric Association Task Force (1991) Quantitative electroencephalography: A report on the present state of computerized EEG techniques. American Journal of Psychiatry **148**, 961–964.

Anonymous, (1993) The tenth annual directory of medical hardware and software companies. MD Computing **10**, 231–267.

Arbogast, J. G. and Dodrill, W. H. (1985) Diabetes home monitoring by telephone data entry. Clinics in Primary Care **12**, 573–579.

Arenson, R. L., Chakraborty, D. P., Seshadri, S. B. and Kindel, H. L. (1990) The digital imaging workstation. Radiology **176**, 303–315.

Bachorik, P. S. (1987) Lipid profile consultation. MD Computing **4**, 50–52.

Baechtel, F. S., Monson, K. L., Forsen, G. E., Budowle, B. and Kearney, J. J. (1991) Tracking the violent criminal offender through DNA typing profiles – a national database system concept. Experientia **58**, 356–360.

Baker, P. G. (1987) Author Languages for CAL. Macmillan Education, London.

Bakker, A. R. (1990) An integrated hospital information system in the Netherlands. Clinical Computing **7**, 91–97.

Ball, M. J., Warnock-Materon, A., Hannah, K. J. and Douglas, J. V. (1986) The case for using computers in the operating room. Western Journal of Medicine **145**, 843–847.

Bankowitz, R. A., McNeil, M. A., Challinor, S. M., Parker, R. C., Kapoor, W. N. and Miller, R. A. (1989) A computer-assisted medical diagnostic consultation service. Annals of Internal Medicine **110**, 824–832.

Banks, G., Vries, J. K. and McLinden, S. (1987) Radiologic automated diagnosis (RAD). Computer Methods and Programs in Biomedicine **15**, 157–168.

Barlow, P., Murray, G. D. and Teasdale G. (1987) Outcome after severe head injury: the Glasgow model. In: Medical Applications of Microcomputers (ed. Corbett, W. A.), Wiley, New York, pp. 105–126.

Barnard, G. W., Robbins, L., Tingle, D., Shaw, T. and Newman G. (1987) Development of a computerized sexual assessment laboratory. Bulletin of the American Society of Psychiatry and Law **15**, 339–347.

Barnett, G. O., Cimino, J. J., Huypp, J. A. and Hoffer, E. P. (1987) An evolving diagnostic decision-support system. Journal of Anerican Medical Association **258**, 67–74.

Barsalov, T. and Brutlag, D. L. (1991) Searching gene and protein sequence databases. MD Computing **8**, 144–149.

Barton, N. (1989) Repetitive strain disorder. British Medical Journal ii, 405–406.

Bennett, A. E. and Ritchie, K. (1975) Questionnaires in Medicine: A Guide to their Design and Use, Oxford University Press, London, New, York, Toronto.

Benson, T. (1991) Medical Informatics, Longman Group Ltd, Harlow.

Bergeron, B. and Locke, S. (1990) Speech recognition as a user interface. MD Computing **7**, 329–333.

Berman, D. A., Coleridge, S. T. and McMurry, E. A. (1989) Computerized algorithm-directed triage in the Emergency Department. Annals of Emergency Medicine **18**, 141–144.

Bernadt, M. W., Daniels, P. J., Blizard, R. A. and Murray, R. M. (1989) Can a computer reliably elicit an alcohol history. British Journal of Addiction **84**, 405–411.

Bernstein, L. M., Siegal, E. R. and Goldstein, C. M. (1980) The hepatitis knowledge base: a prototype information transfer system. Archives of Internal Medicine **93**, 169–175.

Bessette, F. and Nguyen, L. (1989) Automated electrocardiogram analysis: the state of the art. Medical Informatics **14**, 43–51.

Bickers, R. G. (1985) Online medical information services. Clinics in Primary Care **12**, 459–482.

Bickers, R. G. (1985) MEDLINE and Beyond: The Personal Computer Guide to Retrieval and Management of Medical Information, Year Book Medical Publishers, Chicago.

Binik, Y., Westbury, C. F. and Servan-Schreiver, D. (1989) Interaction with a 'Sex-expert' system enhances attitudes towards computerised sex therapy. Behavioural Research and Therapy **27**, 303–306.

Bishop, C. W. (1989) A name is not enough. MD Computing **6**, 200–206.

Black, G. C. and Ashton, A. L. (1985) Health risk appraisal in primary care. Clinics in Primary Care **12**, 557–571.

Blackwell, R. and Chang, A. (1988) Video display terminals and pregnancy: A review. British Journal of Obstetrics and Gynaecology **95**, 446–453.

Blamey, P. J. and Clark, G. M. (1987) Psychophysical studies relevant to the design of a digital electrotactile speech processor. Journal of the Acoustic Society of America **82**, 116–125.

Blamey, P. J., Dowell, R. C., Brown, A. M., Clark, G. M. and Seligman, P. M. (1987b) Vowel and consonant recognition of cochlear implant patients using format-estimating speech processors. Journal of the Acoustic Society of America **81**, 48–57.

Bleich, H. L., Safran, C and Slack, W. V. (1989) Departmental and laboratory computing in two hospitals. MD Computing **6**, 149–155.

Bloch, R., Sweeney, G., Ahmed, K., Dickinson, C. J. and Ingram, D. (1980) MACDOPE: a simulation of drug disposition in the human body. Applications in clinical pharmacokinetics. British Journal of Clinical Pharmacology **10**, 591–602.

Blois, M. S. (1984) Information and Medicine: The Nature of Medical Descriptions, University of California Press, Berkeley.

Boulton, L. M. (1993) Computer hardware and software to assist the visually impaired and blind. Australia and New Zealand Journal of Ophthalmology **21**, 7–14.

Branger, P. J., van der Wouden, J. C., Schudel, B. R., Verboog, E., Duisterhout, J. S., van der Lei, J. and van Bemmel, J. H. (1992) Electronic communication between providers of primary and secondary care. British Medical Journal **305**, 1068–1970.

Brannigan, V. (1987) The regulation of medical computer software as a device under the Food, Drug, and Cosmetic Act. Computer Methods and Programs in Biomedicine **25**, 219–228.

Brannigan, V. M. and Mola, E. C. (1990) Liability exposure for the use of computers in obstetrics and gynecology. In: Computers in Obstetrics and Gynecology (eds Dalton, K. J. and Chard, T), Elsevier Science Publishers BV (Biomedical Division), pp. 287–298.

Broekemeier, R. L., Cooper, C. B., O'Brien, M. S., Munro, M. R. and Giese, R. M. (1986) Implementing a stand-alone packaged pharmacy computer system in a 580-bed hospital. American Journal of Hospital Pharmacy **43**, 653–658.

Brownbridge, G., Herzmark, G. A. and Wall, T. D. (1985) Patient reactions to doctors' computer use in general practice consultations. Science and Medicine **20**, 47–52.

Bruns, B. J. (1991) Productivity enhancements using hand-held computers: A case study. Biomedical Instrumentation and Technology, March/April, 122–128.

Brusco, M. J., Futch, J. and Showalter, M. J. (1993) Nurse staff planning under conditions of a nursing shortage. Journal of Nursing Administration **23**, 58–64.

Burger, R. E., Frost, C. D. and Dalton, K. J. (1987) Computerized ultrasonic image analysis for placental characterization in normal and hypertensive pregnancies. International Journal of Biomedical Computing **21**, 95–111.

Camma, C., Garofalo, G., Almasio, P., Tine, F., Craxi, A., Palazzo, U., Pinzello, G. B., Fiorello, F., Angelo, P. M. and Pagliaro, L. (1991) A performance evaluation of the expert system 'Jaundice' in comparison with that of three hepatologists. Journal of Hepatology **13**, 279–285.

Chan, L. S. and Portnoy, B. (1988) Evaluation of statistical packages for suitability for use by clinical investigators in medicine. Computer Methods and Programs in Biomedicine **27**, 83–94.

Chang, R. W., Lee, B. and Jacobs, S. (1989) Accuracy of decisions to withdraw therapy in critically ill patients: clinical judgement versus a computer model. Critical Care Medicine **17**, 1091–1097.

Chao, A. K. H. and Chao, T. C. (1990) Computer graphics in medical illustration. Annals Academy of Medicine of Singapore **19**, 745–751.

Chapman, C. M., Miller, J. G., Bruenger, J. A., Wysor, W. J., Meininger, E. T., Wolf, F. M., Fischer, T. V., Beaudoin, A. R. and Birkel, W. E. (1992) ATLAS-plus: multimedia instruction in embryology, gross anatomy, and histology. In: Proceedings of the Annual Symposium on Computer Applications in Medical Care, 712–716.

Chard, T. (1987a) Self-learning for a Bayesian knowledge base: how long does it take for the machine to educate itself? Methods of Information in Medicine **26**, 185–188.

Chard, T. (1987b) Human versus machine: a comparison of a computer 'expert system' with human experts in the diagnosis of vaginal discharge. International Journal of Biomedical Computing **20**, 71–78.

Chard, T. (1989a) The effect of dependence on the performance of Bayes theorem: an evaluation using a computer simulation. Computer Methods and Programs in Biomedicine **29**, 15–19.

Chard, T. and Rubenstein, E. M. (1989b) A model-based system to determine the relative value of different variables in a diagnostic system using Bayes theorem. International Journal of Biomedical Computing **24**, 133–142

Chard, T. (1990a) Computers and Preinatal Medicine. In: Proceedings of 2nd World Symposium 'Computers in the Care of the Mother, Fetus and Newborn' (eds Maeda, K., Hogaki, M. and Nakano, H.), Excerpta Medica, Kyoto, pp. 27–36.

Chard, T. (1990b) An Introduction to Radioimmunoassay and Related Techniques, Elsevier, Amsterdam, New York, London.

Chard, T. and Schreiner, A. (1990c) Expert Systems in obstetrics and gynaecology. Baillière's Clinical Obstetrics and Gynaecology **4**, 815–840

Chard, T. (1991) Qualitative probability versus quantitative probability in clinical diagnosis. Medical Decision Making **11**, 38–41.

Cimino, J. J. and Barnett, G. O. (1990) Automated translation between medical terminologies using semantic definitions. MD Computing **7**, 104–109.

Cimino, J. J., Johnson, S. B., Aguirre, A., Roderer, N. and Clayton, P. D. (1992) The Medline Button, in Fifteenth Annual Symposium on Computer Applications in Medical Care (ed. Clayton, P. D.), McGraw-Hill, Baltimore, pp. 81–85.

Clarke, J. R., Cebula, D. P. and Webber, B. L. (1988) Artificial intelligence: a computerized decision aid for trauma. The Journal of Trauma **28**, 1250–1253.

Classen, D. C., Pestonik, S. L., Evans, R. S. and Burke, J. P. (1991) Computerized surveillance of adverse drug events in hospital patients. Journal of the American Medical Association **266**, 2847–2851.

Clayden, G. S. and Wilson, B. (1988) Computer-assisted learning in medical education. Medical Education **22**, 456–467.

Clyman, S. G., Julian, E. R., Orr, N. A., Dillon, G. F. and Cotton, K. E. (1992) Continued research on computer-based testing. In: Fifteenth Annual Symposium on Computer Applications in Medical Care (ed. Clayton, P. D.), McGraw-Hill, New York, pp. 742–746.

Cobb, H. (1986) Computer applications in veterinary medical education. Veterinary Clinics in North America **16**, 703–708.

Coleman, T. G. and Randal, J. E. (1983) Human, a comprehensive physiological model. Physiologist **26**, 15–21.

Comhaire, F. H., Huysse, S., Hinting, A., Vermeulen, L. and Schoonjans, F. (1992) Objective semen analysis: has the target been reached? Human Reproduction **7**, 237–241.

Connelly, D. P. and Willard, K. E. (1989) Monte Carlo simulation and the clinical laboratory. Archives of Pathology and Laboratory Medicine **113**, 750–757

Connelly, D. P. and Bennett, S. T. (1991) Expert systems and the clinical laboratory information system. Laboratory and Hospital Information Systems **11**, 125–151.

Cook, V. and McCorkel, J. (1987) Computer-assisted instruction for medicine and nursing: sources and programs. Bulletin of Medical Librarian Association **75**, 101–108.

Corwin, J. and Snodgrass, J. G. (1987) The picture memory and fragmented pictures tests: use with cognitively impaired population. Psychopharmacology Bulletin **23**, 286–291.

Cote, R. A. and Rothwell, D. J. (1989) The classification nomenclature issues in medicine: a return to natural language. Medical Informatics **14**, 25–41.

Cowan, D. B. and Chard, T. (1985) The perinatal database: content and collection. British Journal of Hospital Medicine **34**, 37–41.

Crevasse, L., Robinson, J. D., Ariet, M. and Sung, J. (1988) A program for optimizing drug dosage regimens: digoxin. MD Computing **5**, 27–34.

Culbert, A. J., Cantelmo, N. L., Stafford, M. E. and Allan, D. M. E. (1989) Interactive videodisc as an instructional tool in medical education. Methods of Information in Medicine **28**, 357–359.

Cutting, C., Grayson, B., Bookstein, F., Fellingham, L. and McCarthy, J. G. (1986) Computer-aided planning and evaluation of facial and orthognathic surgery. Clinical Plastic Surgery **13**, 449–462.

Czaja, S. J. and Sharit, J. (1993) Age differences in the performance of computer-based work. Psychology and Aging **8**, 59–67.

Dalton, K. J. (1990) On-line databases. In: Computers in Obstetrics and Gynaecology (eds Dalton, K. J. and Chard, T.), Elsevier Science Publishers BV (Biomedical Division), pp. 301–311.

Dambro, M. R., Weiss, B. D., McClare, C. L. and Vuturo, A. F. (1988) An unsuccessful experience with computerized medical records in an academic medical center. Journal of Medical Education **63**, 617–623.

Dawkins, R. (1986) Creation and natural selection. New Scientist **18**, 34–38.

de Dombal, F. T., Horrocks, J. C., Staniland, J. R. and Guillou, P. J. (1971) Production of artificial 'case histories' by using a small computer. British Medical Journal **ii**, 578–581.

de Dombal, F. T., Leaper, D. J. K., Horrocks, J. C. and McCann, A. P. (1972) Computer aided diagnosis of acute abdominal pain. British Medical Journal **ii**, 9–13.

Diamond, G. A., Rozanski, A. and Steuer, M. (1986) Playing Doctor: application of game theory to medical decision making. Journal of Chronic Disease **39**, 669–677.

Dickey, R. and Shealey, S. H. (1987) Using technology to control the environment. The American Journal of Occupational Therapy **41**, 717–721.

Dickinson, C. J. (1977) A Computer Model of Human Respiration, MTP Press, Lancaster.

Diserens, D., Schwartz, M. W., Guenin, M. and Taylor, L. A. (1986) Measuring the problem-solving ability of students and residents by microcomputer. Journal of Medical Education **61**, 461–466.

Divon, M. Y. and Boucher, D. R. (1990) Computer-assisted fetal monitoring. In: Computers in Obstetrics and Gynaecology (eds Dalton, K. J. and Chard, T.), Elsevier Science Publishers B.V. (Biomedical Division) Amsterdam, pp. 59–78.

Dolan, J. G., Bodley, D. R. and Mushlin, A. I. (1986) An evaluation of clinicians subjective prior probability estimates. Medical Decision Making **6**, 216–223.

Dooling, S. L. (1987) Designing computer simulations. Computers in Nursing **219**, 224.

Duisterhout, J. S. and Schoemaker, J. (1987) AIDA for reproductive medicine and the fertility clinic. Computer Methods and Programs in Biomedicine **25**, 305–314.

Dytch, H. E. and Wied, G. L. (1990) Artificial neural networks and their use in quantitative pathology. Analytical and Quantitative Cytology and Histology **12**, 379–393.

Ellis, D. (1987) The artificial expert. In: Medical Computing and Applications, Ellis Horwood, Chichester, pp. 81–117.

Elstein, A. S., Kaga, N., Shulman, L. S., Jason, H. and Loupe, M. (1972) Methods and theory in the study of medical enquiry. Journal of Medical Education **47**, 85–92.

Elstein, A., Shulman, L. and Sprafka, S. (1978) Medical Problem Solving: An Analysis of Clinical Reasoning, Harvard University Press, Cambridge, MA.

Erdman, H. P., Klein, M. H. and Greist, J. H. (1985) Direct patient computer interviewing. Journal of Consulting and Clinical Psychology **53**, 760–773.

Evans, S. (1985) Computer literacy in family medicine. Clinics in Primary Care **12**, 403–413.

Feinstein, A., Rubenstein, J. and Ramshaw, W. (1972) Estimating prognosis with the aid of a conversational-mode computer program. Annals of Internal Medicine **76**, 911–921.

Fenyo, G. (1990) Computer-aided diagnosis and decision-making in acute abdominal pain. Digestive Diseases and Sciences **8**, 125–137.

Feskanich, D., Buzzard, I. M., Welch, B. T., Asp, E. H., Dieleman, L. S., Chong, K. R. and Bartsch, G. E. (1988) Comparison of a computerized and manual method of food coding for nutrient intake studies. Journal of American Dietetic Association **88**, 1263–1267.

First, M. B., Soffer, L. J. and Miller, R. A. (1985) QUICK (Quick Index to Caduceus Knowledge): using the Internist-1/Caduceus knowledge base as an electronic textbook of medicine. Computers and Biomedical Research **18**, 137–165.

First, M. B., Opler, L. A., Hamilton, R. M., Linder, J., Linfield, L. S., Silver, J. M., Toshav, N. L., Kahn, D., Williams, D. B. and Spitzer, R. L. (1993) Evaluation in an inpatient setting of DTREE, a computer-assisted diagnostic assessment procedure. Comprehensive Psychiatry **34**, 171–175.

Fisher, L. A., Johnson, T. S., Porter, D., Bleich, H. L. and Slack, W. V. (1977) Collection of a clean voided urine specimen: a comparison among spoken, written and computer-based instructions. American Journal of Public Health **67**, 640–644.

Fowler, R. D. (1985) Landmarks in computer-assisted psychological assessment. Journal of Consulting Clinical Psychology **53**, 748–759.

Franke, R., Huebel, S. and Streich, W. J. (1985) Substructural QSAR approaches and topological pharmacophores. Environmental Health Perspective **61**, 239–255.

Franklin, R. C. G., Spiegelhalter, D. J., Macartney, F. J. and Bull, K. (1991) Evaluation of a diagnostic algorithm for heart disease in neonates. British Medical Journal **302**, 935–939.

French, C. C. and Beaumont, J. G. (1987) The reaction of psychiatric patients to computerized assessment. British Journal of Clinical Psychology **26**, 267–278.

Friede, A., Reid, J. A. and Ory, H. W. (1993) CDC WONDER: a comprehensive on-line public health information system of the Centers for Disease Control and

Prevention. American Journal of Public Health **83**, 1289–1294.

Friedman, R. H. (1986) The use of computers to assist physicians in patient management. In: Annual Review of Medicine, Year Book Medical Publishers, Chicago.

Frisse, M. E. (1990) The case for hypermedia. Academic Medicine **6**, 17–19.

Fryback, D. G. (1986) A program for training and feedback about probability estimation for physicians. Computer Methods and Programs in Biomedicine **22**, 27–33.

Furfine, C. S. (1992) The FDA's policy on the regulation of computerized medical devices. MD Computing **9**, 97–100.

Gammerman, G. E. (1992) FDA regulation of biomedical software. Proceedings of the Annual Symposium on Computer Applications in Medical Care 745–749. (Abstract).

Garrett, T. J., Ashford, A. R. and Savage, D. G. (1987) A comparison of computer-assisted instruction and tutorials in hematology and oncology. Journal of Medical Education **62**, 918–922.

Gell, G. (1993) Expert systems as a support for radiological diagnosis. European Journal of Radiology **17**, 8–13.

Gibbons, R. D. and Fiedler-Weiss, V. C. (1986) Computer-aided quantification of scalp hair. Dermatology Clinics **4**, 627–640.

Gilpin, E. A., Olshen, R. A., Chatterjee, K., Kjekshus, J., Moss, A. J., Henning, H., Engler, R., Blacky, A. R., Dittrich, H. and Ross, J. (1990) Predicting 1-year outcome following acute myocardial infarction: physicians versus computers. Computers and Biomedical Research **23**, 46–63.

Gitlin, J. N. (1986) Teleradiology. Radiology Clinics of North America **24**, 55–68.

Goh, J. C. H., Ho, N. C. and Bose, K. (1990) Principles and applications of computer-aided design and computer-aided manufacturing (CAD/CAM) technology in orthopaedics. Annals of the Academy of Medicine Singapore **19**, 706–712.

Golden, W. E. and Friedlander, I. R. (1987) Inverse technology and medical education. Lancet **i**, 851–853.

Goldman, B. (1990) Advanced clinical problems on disk: a software review. Candian Medical Association Journal **142**, 1122–1123.

Goldman, L., Cook, E. F., Brand, D. A., Lee, T. H., Rouan, G. W., Weisberg, M. C., Acampora, D., Stasiulewicz, C., Walshon, J., Terranova, G., Gottlieb, L., Kobernick, M., Goldstein-Wayne, B., Copen, D., Daley, K., Brandt, A. A., Jones, D., Mellors, J. and Kakubowski, R. (1988) A computer protocol to predict myocardial infarction in emergency department patients with chest pain. New England Journal of Medicine **318**, 797–803.

Gonzalez, F. A. and Fox, H. E. (1989) The development and implementation of a computerized on-line obstetric record. British Journal of Obstetrics and Gynaecology **96**, 1323–1327.

Gordon, C. (1991) Supporting acts. British Journal of Healthcare Computing **9**, 29–30.

Gosney, M. and Tallis, R. C. (1984) Prescription of contraindicated and interacting drugs in elderly patients admitted to hospital. Lancet **i**, 564–567.

Gould, J. D., Alfaro, L., Banres, V., Finn, R., Grischowsky, N. and Minuto, A. (1987) Reading is slower from CRT displays than from paper: Attempts to isolate a single-variable explanation. Human Factors **29**, 269–299.

Gouveia, W. A. (1986) Computer lessons relearned. American Journal of Hospital Pharmacy **43**, 614.

Grams, R. R. and Jin, Z. M. (1989) The natural language processing of medical databases. Journal of Medical Systems **13**, 79.

Green, M. (1986) The Psion organizer for Community data collection. British Journal of Healthcare Computing **2**, 36.

Greenes, R. A. and Shortliffe, E. H. (1990) Medical Informatics: an emerging academic discipline and institutional priority. Journal of the American Medical Association **263**, 1114–1120.

Griffiths, P. D., Green, A., Platt, P., Morris, J. and Assheton, J. (1987) Neonatal blood screening. British Journal of Healthcare Computing **44**, 34–35.

Gustafson, D. H., Bosworth, K., Hawkins, R. P., Boberg, E. W. and Bricker, E. (1992) CHESS: a computer-based system for providing information, referrals, decision support and social support to people facing medical and other health-related crises, in Fifteenth Annual Symposium on Computer Applications in Medical Care (ed. Clayton, P. D.), McGraw-Hill, Baltimore, pp. 161–165.

Guy, J. F. and Frisby, A. J. (1992) Using interactive videodiscs to teach gross anatomy to undergraduates at the Ohio State University. Academic Medicine **67**, 132–133.

Hall, G. C., Luscombe, D. K. and Walker, S. R. (1988) Post-marketing surveillance using a computerised general practice data base. Pharmaceutical Medicine **2**, 345–351.

Hancock, D. M., Heptinsall, M., Old, J. M., Lobo, F. X., Contractor, B. R., Chaturvedi, S., Chan, M. and de Dombal, F. T. (1987) Computer aided diagnosis of acute abdominal pain. The practical impact of a 'theoretical' exercise. Theoretical Surgery **2**, 99–105.

Hardman, L. (1990) Introduction to Hypertext and Hypermedia. Education **9**, 2–11.

Harkin, P. J. R., Dixon, M. F., Reid, W. A. and Bird, C. C. (1986) Computer assisted learning systems in pathology teaching. Medical Teacher **8**, 27–34.

Harless, W. G., Zier, M. A. and Toothman, J. P. (1985) Technological Innovations in Medical Education. The TIME Project. In: Proceedings of the Symposium on Computer Applications in Medical Care (SCAMC), pp. 596–597.

Harris, R. P., O'Malley, M. S., Fletcher, S. W. and Knight, B. P. (1990) Prompting physicians for preventive procedures: a five-year study of manual and computer reminders. American Journal of Preventive Medicine **6**, 145–151.

Hashimoto, D., Dohi, T., Tszuki, M., Horiuchi, T., Ohta, Y., Chinzei, K., Suzuki, M. and Idezuki, Y. (1991) Development of a computer-aided surgery system: Three-dimensional graphic reconstruction for treatment of liver cancer. Surgery **109**, 589–596.

Hasman, A. (1982) Training in medical informatics. The use of computers for diagnostic purposes. International Journal of Biomedical Computing **13**, 109–118.

Haug, P. J., Warner, H. R., Clayton, P. D., Schmidt, C. D., Pearl, J. E., Farney, R. J., Crapo, R. O., Tocino, I., Morrison, W. J. and Frederick, P. R. (1987) A decision-driven system to collect the patient history. Computers in Biochemical Research **20**, 207–211.

Haumschild, M. J., Ward, E. S., Bishop, J. M. and Haumschild, M. S. (1987) Pharmacy-based computer system for monitoring and reporting drug interactions. American Journal of Hospital Pharmacy **44**, 345–348.

Hauser, T., Kraegen, E. W., Campgell, L. V., Compton, P. J., Sammut, C. and Chisholm, D. J. (1992) Assessment of experts' approach to insulin therapy and development of a simulator for diabetes insulin adjustment. Diabetes Care **15**, 221–231.

Haynes, R. B., McKibbon, K. A., Walker, C. J. and Mosseau, J. (1985) Computer searching of the medical literature. Annals of Internal Medicine **103**, 812–816.

Haynes, R. B. and Walker, C. J. (1987) Computer aided quality assurance. A critical appraisal. Archives of Internal Medicine **147**, 1297–1301.

Haynes, R. B., McKibbon, K. A., Bayley, E., Walker, C. J. and Johnston, M. E. (1992) Increases in knowledge and use of information technology by entering medical students at McMaster University in successive annual surveys, in Fifteenth Annual Symposium on Computer Applications in Medical Care (ed. Clayton, P. D.), McGraw-Hill, Baltimore, pp. 560–563.

Heathfield, H. A. and Wyatt, J. (1993) Philosophies for the design and development of clinical decision-support systems. Methods of Information in Medicine **32**, 1–8.

Heizmann, W., Pickert, A., Kloss, T. and Werner, H. (1988) New developments in medical microbiology: computer-assisted diagnosis and automated instruments. Infection **16**, 69–74.

Henderson, J. V. and Black, C. (1980) Computer-assisted diagnosis in acute abdominal pain. US Navy Medicine **7**, 2–4.

Henderson, J. V., Pruett, R. K., Galper, A. R. and Copes, W. S. (1986) Interactive videodisc to teach combat trauma life support. Journal of Medical Systems **10**, 271–276.

Hersh, W. R. and Greenes, R. A. (1990) Information retrieval in medicine: state of the art. MD Computing **7**, 302–309.

Hindel, J. (1990) The impact of image storage organization on the effectiveness of PACS. Journal of Digital Imaging **3**, 205–210.

Hofer, P. J. and Green, B. F. (1985) The challenge of competence and creativity in computerized psychological testing. Journal of Consulting and Clinical Psychology **53**, 826–838.

Howard, A. E. and Kollman, P. A. (1988) An analysis of current methodologies for conformational searching for complex molecules. Journal of Medicinal Chemistry **31**, 1670–1675.

Hripesak, G., Clayton, P. D., Prior, T. A., Haug, P., Wigertz, O. B. and van der Lei, J. (1991) Arden syntax for medical logic modules. MD Computing **8**, 76–78.

Huang, H. K. (1987) Progress in image processing technology related to radiological sciences: a five-year review. Computer Methods and Progress in Biomedicine **25**, 143–156.

Hubbard, S. M., Henney, J. E. and DeVita, V. T. (1987) A computer data base for information on cancer treatment. The New England Journal of Medicine **316**, 315.

Humphreys, B. L. and Lindberg, D. A. (1993) The UMLS project: making the conceptual connection between users and the information they need. Bulletin of Medical Librarian Association **81**, 170–177

Inaraja, M. T., Paloma, J. M., Giraldez, J. and Hualde, S. (1986) Computer-assisted antimicrobial-use monitoring. American Journal of Hospital Pharmacy **43**, 664–670.

Jacky, J. (1989) Programmed for disaster: Software errors that imperil lives. The Sciences **29**, 22–27.

Jelovsek, F. R. (1988) Computer competency program for medical students and residents. AAMSI News **5**, 11–12.

Johnson, J. H. and Williams, T. A. (1980) Using on-line computer technology in a mental health admitting system. In: Technology in Mental Health Care Delivery Systems (eds Sidowski, J. B., Johnson, J. A. and Williams, T. A), Ablex, Norwood, NJ, pp. 237–249.

Johnson, K., Poon, A., Shiffman, S., Lin, R. and Fagan, L. (1992) A history-taking system that uses continuous speech recognition. In: Fifteenth Annual Symposium on Computer Applications in Medical Care (ed. Clayton, P. D.) McGraw-Hill, Baltimore, pp. 757–761

Jones, R. B. and Hedley, A. J. (1986) A computer in the diabetic clinic. Practical Diabetes **3**, 295–296.

Jones, R. B. and Hedley, A. J. (1989) Methods of estimating losses to follow-up from a diabetic clinic. Practical Diabetes **6**, 129–133.

Jones, R. G. (1993) Personal computer software for handling references from CD-ROM and mainframe sources for scientific and medical reports. British Medical Journal **307**, 180–184.

Joseph, L. S. and Joseph, A. F. (1985) Developing educational software for publisher vendors. Nursing Clinics of North America **20**, 529–547.

Jost, R. G., Rodewald, S. S. and Hill, R. L. (1982) A computer system to monitor radiology department activity: a management tool to improve patient care. Radiology **145**, 357–360.

Joyce, E. (1987) Software bugs: a matter of life and liability. Datamation **33**, 88–92.

Kassirer, J. P., Moskowitz, A. J. and Pauker, S. G. (1987) Decision analysis: a progress report. Annals of Internal Medicine **106**, 275–291.

Kellett, J. G. and O'Riordan, J. (1994) A thrombolytic decision tree. MD Computing **167**, 164.

Kennedy, R. L., Harrison, R. F. and Marshall, S. J. (1993) Do we need computer-based decision support for the diagnosis of acute chest pain: discussion paper. Journal of the Royal Society of Medicine **86**, 31–34.

Kerlin, B. D. (1986) Dissemination of COSTAR: promises and realities. Journal of Medical Systems **10**, 265–269.

Kilgallon, M. J., Roberts, D. P. and Miller, S. (1987) Adapting personal computers for use by high-level quadriplegics. Medical Instrumentation **21**, 97–102.

Kilpatrick, K. E., Vogel, W. B. and Carswell, J. L. (1988) Evolution of a computerized support system for health care capacity planning. Journal of Medical Systems **12**, 305–317.

Kiuru, A., Akisada, M., Okabe, T., Olsson, S. and Saranummi, N. (1991) PACS in Japan and the Nordic Countries: First Japan-Nordic PACS Symposium. Computer Methods and Progress in Biomedicine **36**, 65–70.

Kleinmuntz, B. and Elstein, A. S. (1987) Computer modelling of clinical judgement. Critical Reviews in Medical Informatics **1**, 209–227.

Klopman, G. (1985) Predicting toxicity through a computer automated structure evaluation program. Environmental Health Perspective **61**, 269–274.

Knill-Jones, R. P., Stern, R. B., Grimes, D. H., Maxwell, J. D., Thompson, R. P. H. and Williams, R. (1973) Use of a sequential Bayesian model in the diagnosis of jaundice. British Medical Journal **i**, 530–533.

Kors, J. A., Sittig, A. C. and van Bemmel, J. H. (1990) The Delphi method to validate diagnostic knowledge in computerized ECG interpretation. Methods of Information in Medicine **29**, 44–50.

Kruse, K. A. (1986) Building a practice with a computer. Veterinary Journal of North America **16**, 723–729.

Kurlychek, R. T. and Levin, W. (1988) Computers in the cognitive rehabilitation of brain-injured persons. Critical Review in Medical Informatics **1**, 241–257.

Laidlaw, J. M. (1989) Twelve tips for designing instructional text using desktop publishing. Medical Teacher **11**, 139–143.

Lancioni, G. E. and Oliva, D. (1988) A computer-aided programme for promoting unsupervized activities for multihandicapped adolescents. Journal of Mental Deficiency Research **32**, 125–136.

Langlotz, C. P., Shortliffe, E. H. and Fagan, L. M. (1988) A methodology for generating computer-based explanations of decision-theoretic advice. Medical Decision Making **8**, 290–303.

Langton, K. B. Johnston, M. E., Haynes, R. B. and Mathieu, A. (1992) A critical appraisal of the literature on the effects of computer-based clinical decision support systems on clinician performance and patient outcome. In: Fifteenth Annual Symposium on Computer Applications in Medical Care (ed. Clayton, P. D.), McGraw-Hill, Baltimore, pp. 626–630.

Leao, B. F. and Roche, A. F. (1990) Proposed methodology for knowledge acquisition: a study on congenital heart disease. Methods of Information in Medicine **29**, 30–40.

Lee, T. H., Juarez, G., Cook, E. F., Weisberg, M. C., Rouan, G. W., Brand, D. A. and Goldman, L. (1991) Ruling out acute myocardial infarction: a prospective multicenter validation of a 12-hour strategy for patients at low risk. The New England Journal of Medicine **324**, 1239–1246.

Legler, J. D. (1990) Physicians' accuracy in manual computation. MD Computing **7**, 155–159.

Lelliott, P. (1994) Making clinical informatics work. British Medical Journal **308**, 802–803.

Lehky, S. R. and Sejnowski, T. J. (1988) Network model of shape-from-shading: neural function arises from both receptive and projective fields. Nature **333**, 452–454.

Lenert, L. A., Lurie, J., Sheiner, L. B., Klostermann, H. and Blaschke, T. R. (1992) Advanced computer programs for drug dosing that combine pharmacokinetic and symbolic modelling of patients. Computers in Biochemical Research **25**, 29–42.

Leotta, D. F., Rabinowitz, W. M., Reed, C. M. and Durlach, N. I. (1988) Preliminary results of speech-reception tests obtained with the synthetic Tadoma system. Journal of Rehabilitation Research **25**, 45–52.

Levine, J. A., Madden, A. M. and Morgan, M. Y. (1987) Validation of a computer based system for assessing dietary intake. British Medical Journal **295**, 369–372.

Levy, A. H. (1989) Factors affecting computer-mediated instruction in medical education. Methods of Information in Medicine **28**, 215–222.

Liehn, J. C., Hannequin, S., Nasca, S., Lebrun, D., Cattan, A. and Valeyre, J. (1987) A new approach to image subtraction in immunoscintigraphy: Preliminary results. European Journal of Nuclear Medicine **13**, 391–396.

Lilford, R. J., Glyn-Evans, D. and Chard, T. (1983) The use of a patient-interactive microcomputer system to obtain histories in an infertility and gynecologic endocrinology clinic. American Journal of Obstetrics and Gynecology **146**, 374–379.

Lilford, R. J., Kelly, M., Baines, A., Cameron, S., Cave, M., Guthrie, K. and Thornton, J. (1992) Effect of using protocols on medical care: randomised trial of three methods of taking an antenatal history. British Medical Journal **305**, 1181–1184.

Lin, R., Lenert, L., Middleton, B. and Shiffman, S. (1992) A free-text processing system to capture physical findings: canonical phrase identification system (CAPIS). In: Fifteenth Annual Symposium on Computer Applications in Medical Care (ed. Clayton, P. D.), McGraw-Hill, New York, pp. 168–172.

Lincoln, T. L. and Aller, R. D. (1991) Acquiring a laboratory computer system: vendor selection and contracting. Laboratory and Hospital Information Systems **11**, 21–40.

Lindberg, D. A. B., Siegel, E. R., Rapp, B. A., Wallingford, K. T. and Wilson, S. R. (1993) Use of MEDLINE by physicians for clinical problem solving. Journal of the American Medical Association **269**, 3124–3129.

Lindberg, G. (1982) Studies on diagnostic decision making in jaundice, Karolinska Institutet, Stockholm.

Lindberg, G., Thomsen, C., Malchow-Moller, A., Matzen, P. and Hilden, J. (1987) Differential diagnosis of jaundice: applicability of the Copenhagen pocket chart proved in Stockholm patients. Liver **7**, 43–49.

Linnarsson, R. and Wigertz, O. (1989) The Data Dictionary – A controlled vocabulary for integrating clinical databases and medical knowledge bases. Methods of Information in Medicine **28**, 78–85.

Linsker, R. (1986) From basic network principles to neural architecture: Emergence of spatial-opponent cells. Proceedings of the National Academy of Sciences USA **83**, 7508–7512.

Lloyd, S. C. (1985) Developments towards clinical support systems. Clinics in Primary Care **12**, 429–443.

Lloyd, T., Sherrard, M. G., Hulse, S. F., Lingle, V. A. and Burnside, J. W. (1989) Designing and implementing a computer learning center in a college of medicine. Journal of Biocommunications **16**, 2–6.

Lo, S. C., Freedman, M. T., Lin, J. S. and Mun, S. K. (1993) Automatic lung nodule detection using profile matching and back-propagation neural network techniques. Journal of Digital Dialling **6**, 48–54.

Locke, S. E., Kowaloff, H. B., Hoff, R. G., Safran, C., Popovsky, M. A., Cotton, D. J., Finkelstein, D. M., Page, P. L. and Slack, W. V. (1992) Computer-based interview for screening blood donors for risk of HIV transmission. Journal of the American Medical Association **268**, 1301–1305.

Lowry, S. and MacPherson, G. (1988) A blot on the profession. British Medical Journal **296**, 657–658.

Lucas, R. W., Mullins, P. J., Luna, C. B. and McInrry, D. C. (1977) Psychiatrists and a computer as interrogators of patients with alcohol-related illnesses: A comparison. British Journal of Psychiatry **131**, 160–167.

Lynnerup, N. (1993) A computer program for the estimation of time of death. Journal of Forensic Sciences **38**, 816–820.

Maceratini, R., Rafanelli, M., Pisanelli, D. M. and Crollari, S. (1989) Export systems and the pancreatic cancer problem: decision support in the pre-operative diagnosis. Journal of Biomedical Engineering **11**, 487–510.

Macfarlane, P. W. (1990) A brief history of computer-assisted electrocardiography, Methods of Information in Medicine **29**, 272–281.

Malchow-Moller, A., Thomsen, C., Matzen, P., Mindeholm, L., Bjerregaard, B., Bryant, S., Hilden, J., Holst-Christensen, J., Johansen, T. S. and Juhl, E. (1986) Computer diagnosis in jaundice: Bayes' rule founded on 1002 consecutive cases. Journal of Hepatology **3**, 154–163.

Mann, N. H. and Brown, M. D. (1991) Artificial intelligence in the diagnosis of low back pain. Orthopedic Clinics of North America **22**, 303–315.

Mansur, D. J., Blattner, M. M. and Joy, K. I. (1985) Sound graphs: a numerical data analysis method for the blind. Journal of Medical Systems **9**, 163–174.

Marion, R., Niebuhr, B., Petrusa, E. and Weinholtz, D. (1982) Computer-based instruction in basic medical science education. Journal of Medical Education **57**, 521–526.

Marsh, J. L. and Vannier, M. W. (1983) The third dimension in craniofacial surgery. Journal of Plastic Reconstructive Surgery **73**, 759–767.

Marsh, J. L., Vannier, M. W., Bresina, S. and Hemmer, K. M. (1986) Applications of computer graphics in craniofacial surgery. Clinical Plastic Surgery **13**, 441–448.

Martin, D. K. (1991) Making the connection: the VA-Regenstrief Project. Clinical Computing **9**, 91–96.

Martin, Y. C. (1991) Computer-assisted rational drug design. Methods in Enzymology **203**, 587–612.

Matheson, N. W. (1986) Medical libraries and computers: the role of medical libraries in medical informatics. Western Journal of Medicine **145**, 859–863.

McAllister, N. H. (1987) Visual display terminals and operator morbidity. Canadian Journal of Public Health **78**, 62–65.

McCammon, J. A. (1988) Computer-aided molecular design. Science **328**, 486–491.

McDonald, C. J., Hui, S. L. and Smith, D. M. (1984) Reminders to physicians from an introspective computer medical record. Annals of Internal Medicine **100**, 130–138.

McDonald, C. J., Blevins, L., Tierney, W. M. and Martin, D. K. (1988) The Regenstrief medical records. MD Computing **5**, 34–47.

McGovern, K. T. (1994) Applications of virtual reality to surgery. British Medical Journal **308**, 1054–1055.

McIntyre, J. W. R. and Nelson, T. M. (1991) Application of automated human voice delivery to warning devices in an intensive care unit: A laboratory study. International Journal of Clinical Monitoring and Computing **6**, 255–262.

McNutt, R. A. and Selker, H. P. (1988) How did the acute ischemic heart disease predictive instrument reduce unnecessary coronary care unit admissions? Medical Decision Making **8**, 90–94.

Meals, R. A. and Kabo, J. M. (1986) Computerized anatomy instruction. Clinical Plastic Surgery **13**, 816–825.

Meaney, F. J. (1988) Computerized tracing for newborn screening and follow-up: A Review. Journal of Medical Systems **12**, 69–75.

Meier, S. T. and Sampson, J. P. (1989) Use of computer-assisted instruction in the prevention of alcohol abuse. Journal of Drug Education **19**, 245–256.

Meiss, R. A. (1987) Simulated muscles in the teaching laboratory. Academic Computing **2**, 28–46.

Melnick, D. E. (1986) Information technology in evaluation of competence in the health professions. In: Proceedings of the Tenth Annual Symposium on Computer Applications in Medical Care, IEEE Computer Society Press, Washington DC, pp. 191–193.

Michael, J. A. and Rovick, A. A. (1986) Problem-solving in the pre-clinical curriculum: the uses of computer simulations. Medical Teacher 8, 19–25.

Miller, P. L. (1986) Critiquing: A different approach to expert computer advice in medicine. Medical Informatics (London) 11, 29–38.

Miller, R. A., McNeil, M. A., Challinor, S. M., Masari, F. E. and Myers, J. D. (1986) INTERNIST-1/QUICK MEDICAL REFERENCE project: status report. Western Journal of Medicine 145, 816–822.

Miller, R. A., Jamnback, L., Giuse, N. B. and Masarie, F. E. (1992) Extending the capabilities of diagnostic decision support programs through links to bibliographic searching: addition of 'Canned MeSH Logic' to the Quick Medical Reference (QMR) program for use with Grateful Med. In: Fifteenth Annual Symposium on Computer Applications in Medical Care (ed. Clayton, P. D.), McGraw-Hill, New York, pp. 150–155.

Mitchell, J. A., Bridges, A. J., Reid, J. C., Cutts, J. H., Hazelwood, S. and Sharp, G. C. (1992) Preliminary evaluation of learning via the A1?LEARN/Rheumatology Interactive Videodisc System. In: Fifteenth Annual Symposium on Computer Applications in Medical Care (ed. Clayton, P. D.), McGraw-Hill, Baltimore, pp. 169–173.

Moens, H. J. B. and van der Korst, J. (1992) Development and validation of a computer program using Bayes's theorem to support diagnosis of rheumatic disorders. Annals of the Rheumatic Diseases 51, 266–271.

Molteno, B. and Bishop, P. (1986) What CBS means for IT. British Journal of Healthcare Computing 13, 816–825.

Moreland, K. L. (1985) Validation of computer-based test interpretations: problems and prospects. Journal of Consulting and Clinical Psychology 53, 816–825.

Moskowitz, A. J., Kuipers, B. J. and Kassirer, J. P. (1988) Dealing with uncertainty, risks, and tradeoffs in clinical decisions. Annals of Internal Medicine 108, 435–449.

Mugford, M., Banfield, P. and O'Hanlon, M. (1991) Effects of feedback of information on clinical practice: a review. British Medical Journal 303, 398–402.

Mulcahy, D., Mulcahy, R., Reardon, B. and Graham, I. (1986) Can a computer diagnosis of 'normal ECG' be trusted? Irish Journal of Medical Science 155, 416–418.

Mulcahy, D., Reardon, B., Mulcahy, R., Kavanagh, B. and Graham, I. (1986b) Can computer assisted electrocardiography replace a cardiologist for ECG measurements? Irish Journal of Medical Science 155, 410–414.

Mullen, P. D., Carbonari, J. P., Tabak, E. R. and Gleday, M. C. (1991) Improving disclosure of smoking by pregnant women. American Journal of Obstetrics and Gynecology 165, 409–413.

Muller, J. G. and Barash, P. G. (1993) Automated ST-segment monitoring. International Anesthesiology Clinics 31, 45–55.

Murfitt, R. R. (1990) United States Government regulation of medical device software: a review. Journal of Medical Engineering and Technology 14, 111–113.

Nakahara, H., Koyanagi, T., Teraoka, H., Shimokawa, H., Hara, K. and Nakano, H. (1987) Microcomputer-based local area network system for controlling information on perinatal medicine. International Journal of Biomedical Computing 21, 83–93.

O'Connell, W. (1988) Color as a tool for image comparison. MD Computing 5, 14–22.

O'Hara, D. A., Bogen, D. K. and Noordergraaf, A. (1992) The use of computers for controlling the delivery of anesthesia. Anesthesiology 77, 563–581.

Okada, M. (1988) Prolog-based system for nursing staff scheduling implemented on a personal computer. Computers in Biomedical Research 21, 53–63.

Omenn, G. S. and Conrad, D. A. (1984) Implications of DRGs for clinicians. The New England Journal of Medicine 311, 1314–1317.

Osman, L. M., Abdalla, M. I., Beattie, J. A. G., Ross, S. J., Russell, I. T., Friend, J. A., Legge, J. S., Douglas, J. S., on behalf of the Grampian Asthma Study of Integrated Care (GRASSIC). Reducing hospital admission through computer supported education for asthma patients. British Medical Journal 308, 568–571.

Pace, N. L. and Westenskow, D. R. (1983) Computer regulated sodium nitro-prusside infusion for blood pressure control. In: Computing in Anesthesia and Intensive Care (ed. Prakash, O.), Martinus Nijhoff, Boston, pp. 292–301.

Parker, R. C. and Miller, R. A. (1989) Creation of realistic appearing simulated patient cases using the INTERNIST-1/QMR knowledge base and interrelationship properties of manifestations. Methods of Information in Medicine 28, 346–351.

Parsons, D. (1989) Telecommunication discussion groups for health services and medical research. Lancet ii, 1087–1089.

Paterson, C. M., Chapple, J. C., Beard, R. W., Joffe, M., Steer, P. J. and Wright, C. S. W. (1991) Evaluating the quality of maternity services – a discussion paper. British Journal of Obstetrics and Gynaecology 98, 1073–1078.

Pauker, S. G. and Kassirer, J. P. (1987) Decision analysis. The New England Journal of Medicine 316, 250–258.

Pazdernik, T. and Walaszek, E. (1983) A computer-assisted teaching system in pharmacology for health professionals. Journal of Medical Education 58, 341–348.

Pedigo, N. G., Vernon, M. W. and Curry, T. E. (1989) Characterization of a computerized semen analysis system. Fertility and Sterility 52, 659–666.

Peters, M. and Broughton, P. M. G. (1993) The role of expert systems in improving the test requesting patterns of clinicians. Annals of Clinical Biochemistry 30, 52–59.

Peterson, C. M., Jovanic, L. and Chanoch, L. H. (1986) Randomized trial of computer-assisted insulin delivery in patients with Type I diabetes beginning pump therapy. American Journal of Medicine 81, 69–72.

Philip, J. H. (1986) Gas man: an example of goal oriented computer-assisted teaching which results in learning. International Journal of Clinical Monitoring and Computing 3, 165–173.

Pho, R. W. H., Lim, S. Y. E. and Pereira, B. P. (1990) Computer applications in orthopaedics. Annals of the Academy of Medicine Singapore 19, 691–698.

Piemme, T. E. (1988) Computer-assisted learning and evaluation in medicine. Journal of the American Medical Association 260, 367–372.

Pollak, V. E. (1990) Computerized medical information systems enhances quality assurance. Nephron 54, 109–116.

Pollock, R. V. H. (1986) Computers as medical management tools: computer-assisted diagnosis and medical decisions support. Veterinary Journal of North America 16, 669–684.

Poses, R. M., Cebul, R. D. and Centor, R. M. (1988) Evaluating physicians' probabilistic judgments. Medical Decision Making **8**, 233–240.

Prakash, O. (1983) Computing in Anesthesia and Intensive Care, Martinus Nijhoff, Boston.

Prentice, J. W. and Kenny, G. N. C. (1986) Microcomputers in medical education. Medical Teacher **8**, 9–18.

Prinz, P. M., Pemberton, E. and Nelson, K. E. (1985) The ALPHA interactive microcomputer system for teaching, reading, writing and communication skills to hearing-impaired children. American Annals of Deafness **130**, 444–461.

Proost, J. H. and Meijer, D. K. (1992) MW/Pharm, an integrated software package for drug dosage regimen calculation and therapeutic drug monitoring. Computers in Biology and Medicine **22**, 155–163.

Pryor, T. A. (1988) The HELP medical record system. MD Computing **5**, 22–32.

Quaak, M. J., Westerman, R. F. and van Bemmel, J. H. (1987) Comparisons between written and computerised patient histories. British Journal of Medicine **295**, 184–190.

Ratib, O. and Huang, H. K. (1991) Desktop image analysis: workstations of the future. MD Computing **8**, 92–97.

Ray, S. (1985) Computerized language analysis. American Annals of Deafness **130**, 462–469.

Raynor, D. K., Booth, T. G. and Blenkinsopp, A. (1993) Effects of computer generated reminder charts on patients' compliance with drug regimens. British Medical Journal **306**, 1158–1161.

Reggia, J. A. and Tuhrim, S. (1985) Computer-Assisted Medical Decision Making, Springer-Verlag, New York.

Reggia, J. A. (1988) Artificial neural systems in medical science and practice. MD Computing **5**, 4–6.

Rethans, J., Hoppener, P., Wolfs, G. and Diederiks, J. (1988) Do personal computers make doctors less personal? British Medical Journal **296**, 1446–1448.

Richards, J. G. (1984) Computer-assisted instruction and the use of PILOT. Journal of Family Practice **19**, 255–257.

Ritchie, G., Spain, J. and Reves, J. G. (1983) Computer controlled infusion of drugs during anesthesia: method of muscle relaxant and narcotic administration. In: Computing in Anesthesia and Intensive Care (ed. Prakash, O.), Martinus Nijhoff, Boston, pp. 302–315.

Robb, R. A., Hefferman, P. B., Camp, J. J. and Hanson, D. P. (1987) A workstation for multi-dimensional display and analysis of biomedical images. Computer Methods and Progress Biomedicine **25**, 169–184.

Rovick, A. A. and Brenner, L. (1983) Heartsim: a cardiovascular simulation with didactic feedback. Physiologist **26**, 236–239.

Rovick, A. A. and Michael, J. A. (1985) Teaching problem solving in physiology with CBE. Physiologist **28**, 435–438.

Royce, R. (1987) The reality of implementing PAS. British Journal of Healthcare Computing **4**, 14–16.

Rude, F. R. (1986) Computerised medical record keeping. Veterinary Journal of North America **16**, 625–646.

Safran, C., Herrmann, F., Rind, D., Kowaloff, H. B., Bleich, H. L. and Slack, W. V. (1990) Computer-based support for clinical decision making. Clinical Computing **7**, 319–322.

Salyer, K. E., Taylor, D. P. and Billmire, D. E. (1986) Three-dimensional CAT scan reconstruction: pediatric patients. Clinical Plastic Surgery **13**, 463–474.

Sattler, P. W. and Hilburn, L. R. (1985) A program for calculating genetic distance, and its use in determining significant differences in genetic similarity between two groups of populations. Journal of Heredity **76**, 400.

Saudek, C. D., Selam, J.-L., Pitt, H. A., Waxman, K., Rubio, M., Jeandidier, N., Turner, D., Fischell, R. E. and Charles, M. A. (1989) A preliminary trial of the programmable implantable medication system for insulin delivery. The New England Journal of Medicine **321**, 574–579.

Schakel, S. F., Sievert, Y. A. and Buzzard, M. (1988) Sources of data for developing and maintaining a nutrient database. Journal of the American Dietetic Association **10**, 1268–1271.

Scherrer, J.-R., Baud, R. H., Hochstrasser, D. and Ratib, O. (1990) An integrated hospital information system in Geneva. Clinical Computing **7**, 81–88.

Schindler, R. A. and Mezenich, M. M. (1985) Cochlear Implants, Raven, New York.

Schindler, R. A., Kessler, D. K. and Haggerty, H. S. (1993) Clarion cochlear implant: phase I investigational results [corrected; erratum to be published]. American Journal of Otology **14**, 263–272.

Schmiedl, U. P. and Rowberg, A. H. (1990) Literature review: Picture archiving and communication systems. Journal of Digital Imaging **3**, 178–194.

Schneider, S. J., Walter, R. and O'Donnell, R. (1990) Computerised communication as a medium for behavioral smoking cessation treatment: controlled evaluation. Computers and Human Behaviour **6**, 141–151.

Schreiner, A. and Chard, T. (1990) Expert systems for the prediction of ovulation: comparison of an expert system shell (Expertech Xi Plus) with a program written in a traditional language (BASIC). Methods of Information in Medicine **29**, 140–145.

Schreiner, A. and Chard, T. (1991) Some observations on the development of a 'scoring system' in an expert system for prediction of ovulation. International Journal of Biomedical Computing **29**, 245–255.

Schrenck, D. M., Zacharias, D. and Grunau, C. F. V. (1986) Diagnosis of complex acid-base disorders: physician performance versus the microcomputer. Annals of Emergency Medicine **15**, 164–170.

Schultz, E. K., Bauman, A., Hayward, M., Rodbard, D. and Holzman, R. (1992) Improved diabetic prognosis following telecommunication and graphical processing of diabetic data. In: Fifteenth Annual Symposium on Computer Applications in Medicine (ed. Clayton, P. D.), McGraw-Hill, New York, pp. 53–57.

Schwartz, P. W., Patil, R. S. and Szolovits, P. (1986) Artificial intelligence: where do we stand? The New England Journal of Medicine **316**, 685–688.

Scialli, A. R. (1988) A computerized consultation service in Reproductive Toxicology: Summary of the first five years. Obstetrics and Gynecology **72**, 195–199.

Sear, A. M. (1988) An expert system for determining Medicaid eligibility. Journal of Medical Systems **12**, 275–283.

Selmi, P. M., Klein, M. H., Greist, J. H., Sorrell, S. P. and Erdman, H. P. (1991) Computer-administered therapy for depression. MD Computing **8**, 98–102.

Severe, J. B. (1987) Applications of Microcomputers to clinical trials in psychopharmacology. Psychopharmacology Bulletin **23**, 259–260.

Shami, S. (1988) Computerised total parenteral nutrition. In: Microcomputers in

Medicine (eds Coleridge Smith, P. D. and Scurr, J. H.). Springer-Verlag, London, Berlin, Heidelberg, New York, pp. 173–192.

Sharples, S. (1991) DRGs and computing. British Journal of Healthcare Computing **4**, 27–31.

Shortliffe, E (1991) Greek tragedy. British Journal of Healthcare Computing **11**, 13–14.

Siegel, J. H. and Colman, B. (1986) Computers in the care of the critically ill. Urology Clinics of North America **13**, 101–117.

Simons, A. J. R. and Pronk, R. A. F. (1983) Automatic EEG monitoring during anesthesia. In: Computing in Anesthesia and Intensive Care (ed. Prakash, O.), Martinus Nijhoff, Boston, pp. 227–257.

Sivaloganathan, S. (1987) Computers in forensic medicine. Medical Science and Law **27**, 269–279.

Skiba, D. J. (1985) Interactive computer experiences: the missing ingredient. Nursing Clinics of North America **20**, 577–584.

Slack, W. V. and Van Cura, L. J. (1968) Patient reaction to computer-based medical interviewing. Computers in Biomedical Research **1**, 527–531.

Slack, W. V., Leviton, A., Bennett, S. E., Fleischmann, K. H. and Lawrence, R. S. (1988) Relation between age, education and time to respond to questions in a computer-based medical interview. Computers and Biomedical Research **21**, 78–84.

Slack, W. V., Porter, D., Balkin, P., Kowaloff, H. B. and Slack, C. W. (1990) Computer-assisted soliloquy as an approach to psychotherapy. MD Computing **7**, 37–42.

Slovic, P. (1987) Perception of risk. Science **236**, 280–285.

Smith, M. A., Green, S. A., Kuykendall, V. G. and Baum, J. D. (1985) Memory blood glucose reflectance meter and computer: a preliminary report of its use in recording and analysing blood glucose data measured at home by diabetic children. Diabetic Medicine **312**, 924.

Smith, W. J. (1988) Viewing computer color images for medical applications. MD Computing **5**, 58–70.

Sohn, N. and Robbins, R. D. (1985) Computer-assisted surgery. The New England Journal of Medicine **312**, 925.

Sorrell, S. P., Greist, J. H., Klein, M. H., Johnson, J. H. and Harris, W. G. (1982) Enhancement of adherence to tricyclic antidepressants by computerised supervision. Behavioural Research Methods and Instruments **14**, 176–180.

Spencer, I. and Sampson, C. M. (1992) A guide to the use of electronic bulletin boards. Annals of the Royal College of Surgeons of England **74**, 9–13.

Stead, W. W. and Hammond, W. E. (1988) Computer-based medical records: the centerpiece of TMR. MD Computing **5**, 48–62.

Stephens, P. J. and Doherty, J. A. (1992) The use of Apple Macintosh computers and Hypercard in teaching physiology laboratories. American Journal of Physiology **263**, S23–S28

Stigsby, B., Nielsen, P. V. and Docker, M. (1986) Computer description and evaluation of cardiotocograms: a review. Europeran Journal of Obstetrics and Gynecology and Reproductive Biology **21**, 61–86.

Strikeleather, J., Hensel, J. S. and Baumgarten, S. A. (1988) The computerized dental office of the future. Dental Clinics of North America **32**, 173–190.

Stokes, A. V. (1990) Computer communications. In: Computers in Obstetrics and

Gynecology (eds Dalton, K. J. and Chard, T.). Elsevier, Amsterdam, New York, Oxford, pp. 21–31.

Stubbs, D. F. (1988) Neurocomputers. MD Computing **5**, 14–24.

Suenmondt, H. J. and Cooper, G. F. (1992) An evaluation of explanations of probabilistic inference. In: Fifteenth Annual Symposium on Computer Applications in Medical Care (ed. Clayton, P. D.), McGraw-Hill, Baltimore, pp. 579–585.

Sutton, G. C. (1989) Computer-aided diagnosis: a review. British Journal of Surgery **76**, 82–85.

Swank, R. T., Becker, D. M. and Jackson, C. A. (1988) The cost of employee smoking: A computer simulation of hospital nurses. Archives of Internal Medicine **48**, 445–448.

Szolovits, P., Patil, R. S. and Schwartz, W. B. (1988) Artificial intelligence in medical diagnosis. Annals of Internal Medicine **108**, 80–87.

Tallis, R. (1987) Computerised prescribing. In: Medical Applications of Microcomputers (ed. Corbett, W. A.), Wiley, New York, pp. 87–104.

Tate, K. E., Gardner, R. M. and Weaver, L. K. (1990) A computerized laboratory alerting system. MD Computing **7**, 296–301.

Theodoropoulos, G., Loumos, V. and Fillipakis, V. (1993) A multimedia relational database program for parasite identification. Computer Methods and Progress in Biomedicine **39**, 297–301.

Thomas, A. M. C., Fairbank, J. C. T., Pynsent, P. B. and Baker, D. J. (1989) A computer-based interview system for patients with back pain: A validation study. Spine **14**, 844–846.

Tierney, W. M., McDonald, C. J., Hui, S. L. and Martin, D. K. (1988) Computer predictions of abnormal test results: Effects on outpatient testing. Journal of the American Medical Association **259**, 1194–1198.

Tierney, W. M., Miller, M. E. and McDonald, C. J. (1990) The effect of test ordering on informing physicians of the charges for outpatient diagnostic tests. The New England Journal of Medicine **322**, 1499–1504.

Titterington, D. M., Murray, G. D., Murray, L. S., Spiegelhalter, D. J., Skene, A. M., Habbema, J. D. F. and Gelpke, G. J. (1981) Comparison of discrimination techniques applied to a complex data set of head injured patients. Journal of the Royal Statistical Society A, **2**, 145–174.

Treviranus, J. and Tannock, R. (1987) A scanning computer access system for children with severe physical disabilities. American Journal of Occupational Therapy **41**, 733–738.

Tullis, T. S. (1983) The formatting of alphanumeric displays: a review and analysis. Human Factors **25**, 657–682.

Turner, C. W., Lincoln, M. J., Haug, P., Williamson, J. W., Jessen, S., Cundick, K. and Warner, H. (1992) Iliad training effects: a cognitive model and empirical finding. In: Fifteenth Annual Symposium on Computer Applications in Medical Care (ed. Clayton, P. D.), McGraw-Hill, New York, pp. 68–72.

Underhill, L. H. and Bleich, H. L. (1986) Bringing the medical literature to physicians: self service computerised bibliographic retrieval. Western Journal of Medicine **145**, 853–858.

Utsch, M. and Ingram, D. (1978) Generator program for computer-assisted instruction: MACGEN. Computer Programs in Biomedicine **17**, 167–174.

van der Lei, J., Musen, M. A., van der Does, E., Mann in'T Veld, A. J. and van Bemmel, J. H. (1991) Comparison of computer-aided and human review of general practitioners' management of hypertension. Lancet **338**, 1504–1507.

van Gunsteren, W. F. (1988) The role of computer simulation techniques in protein engineering. Protein Engineering **2**, 5–13.

van Mastrigt, R. and Krasne, M. (1993) Automated evaluation of urethral obstruction. Urology **42**, 216–224.

Vandemark, G. J., Kelly, M. and Eckhardt, R. B. (1985) A PASCAL program that calculates heritability estimates using weighted linear regressions. Journal of Heredity **76**, 400–401.

Vozeh, S. (1987) Computer-assisted individualized lidocaine dosage clinical evaluation and comparison with physician performance. American Health Journal **113**, 928–933.

Wain, R. A., Tuhrim, S., D'Autrechy, L. and Reggia, J. A. (1992) The design and automated testing of an expert system for the differential diagnosis of acute stroke. In: Fifteenth Annual Symposium on Computer Applications in Medical Care (ed. Clayton, P. D.), McGraw-Hill, New York, pp. 94–98.

Wald, N. J., Cuckle, H. S., Densem, J. W., Nanchahal, K., Royston, P., Chard, T., Haddow, J. E., Knight, G. J., Palomaki, G. E. and Canick, J. A. (1988) Maternal serum screening for Down's syndrome in early pregnancy. British Medical Journal **297**, 883–887.

Wallin, A. (1993) Interactive quantitative analysis of medical images on a PC- or workstation-based system. Computers in Biology and Medicine **23**, 307–316.

Wallingford, K. T., Humphreys, B. L., Selinger, N. E. and Siegel, E. R. (1990) Bibliographic retrieval: a survey of individual users of Medline. MD Computing **7**, 166–171.

Walsworth-Bell, J. P. and Horseley, S. D. (1988) The use of smart cards in the NHS. Health Trends **20**, 86–88.

Warren, L. (1992) Power, corruption and lies. British Journal of Healthcare Computing **9**, 9–12.

Weaver, R. R. (1991) Assessment and diffusion of computerized decision support systems. International Journal of Technology Assessment Healthcare **7**, 42–50.

Weed, L. L. and Hertzberg, R. (1984) Problem-solving: What's the best combination of man and machine? Computers in Medicine Update **2**, 4–16.

Weilert, M. and Tilzer, L. L. (1991) Putting bar codes to work for improved patient care. Laboratory and Hospital Information Systems **11**, 227–238.

Weiss, S., Kulikowski, C. and Safir A. (1978) Glaucoma consultation by computer. Computers in Biology and Medicine **8**, 25–40.

White, R. (1986) Computer security: an introduction for the medical practitioner. Urology Clinics of North America **13**, 119–128.

White, R. H. (1987) Initiation of warfarin therapy comparison of physician dosing with computer-assisted. Journal of General Internal Medicine **2**, 141–148.

Whiting-O'Keefe, Q. E., Whiting, A. and Henkey, J. (1988) The STOR clinical information system. MD Computing **5**, 8–21.

Wiesel, S. W. and Michelson, L. D. (1986) Monitoring orthopedic patients using computerized algorithms. Orthopedic Clinics of North America **17**, 541–544.

Wigton, R. S., Patel, K. D. and Hoellerich, V. L. (1986) The effect of feedback in learning clinical diagnosis. Journal of Medical Education **61**, 816–822.

Willems, J. L., Arnaud, P., van Bemnel, J. H., Degani, R., Macfarlane, P. W. and Zywietz, C. (1990) Common standards for quantitative electrocardiography: Goals and main results. Methods of Information in Medicine **29**, 263–271.

Willems, J. L., Abreu-Lima, C., Arnaud, P., van Bemmel, H. H., Brohet, C., Degani, R., Denis, B., Gehring, J., Graham, I., van Herpen, G., Machado, H., Macfarlane, P. W., Michaelis, J., Moulopoulos, S. D., Rubel, P. and Zywietz, C. (1991) The diagnostic performance of computer programs for the interpretation of electrocardiograms. The New England Journal of Medicine **325**, 1767–1773.

Wilson, A. L. (1989) Pharma Trend as a management tool: Introduction. American Journal of Hospital Pharmacy **46**, 2009.

Wilson, R. and Crouch, F. A. C. (1987) Risk assessment and comparisons: an introduction. Science **236**, 267–270.

Winkel, P. (1989) The application of expert systems in the clinical laboratory. Clinical Chemistry, **35**, 1595–1600.

Winter, R. M. (1990) Computing and clinical genetics In: Computers in Obstetrics and Gynaecology (eds Dalton, K. J. and Chard, T.), Elsevier Science Publishers B.V. (Biomedical Division), pp. 209–216.

Wong, T. J. and Chua, E. T. (1990) Computers in radiotherapy. Annals of the Academy of Medicine Singapore **19**, 714–719.

Wyatt, J. (1989) Lessons learned from the field trial of ACORN, an expert system to advise on chest pain. In: Proceedings of MEDINFO (Singapore) (eds Manning, P., Zineny, O. and Barber, B.), North Holland, Amsterdam.

Wyatt, J. (1991) Use and sources of medical knowledge. Lancet **338**, 1368–1372.

Wyatt, J. and Spiegelhalter, D. (1992) Field trials of medical decision aids:potential problems and solutions. In: Fifteenth Annual Symposium on Computer Applications in Medical Care (ed. Clayton, P. D.), McGraw-Hill, New York, pp. 3–7.

Xakellis, G. C. and Gjerde, C. (1990) Evaluation by second-year medical students of their computer-aided instruction. Academic Medicine **6**, 23–26.

Yoong, A., Das, S., Carroll, S. and Chard, T. (1993) A national survey to assess current use of computerised information systems in obstetrics. British Journal of Obstetrics and Gynaecology **100**, 205–208.

Yudkin, P. L. and Redman, C. W. G. (1990) Obstetric audit using routinely collected computerised data. British Medical Journal **301**, 1371–1373.

Zadeh, L. (1968) Biological applications of the theory of fuzzy sets and systems. In: Biocybernetics of the Central Nervous System (ed. Proctor, L.), Little Brown and Company, Boston, pp. 199–212.

Zarr, M. L. (1984) Computer-mediated psychotherapy: toward patient selection guidelines. American Journal of Psychology **38**, 1.

Zegher-Geets, I. M., Freeman, A. G., Walker M. G., Blum, R. L. and Wiederhold, G. (1988) Summarization and display of on-line medical records. MD Computing **5**, 38–45.

Index

Note: Page references in *italics* refer to Figures; those in **bold** refer to Tables

Access 10
access to information 66
Activitrax pacemaker 120
adaptive testing 130
administration *see* medical administration
ADONIS 140
Advanced Clinical Problems on Disk 126
ALPHA 116
AMA/GTE Telenet Medical Information
    Network (MINET) 139
AMA/NET 104
ambulatory recording 43
anaesthesia 114
analog signal 38
analog-to-digital conversion 38, *39*
antecedent-driven systems 90
Apple Macintosh computers 1
Apple Macintosh OS 4
appointment systems 24
Arden Syntax 97
array processors 50
arrhythmia monitoring 42
artificial intelligence (AI) 78–9, 94, **94**
artificial perception 79
ASK*MD 96
assembly language 8
audit
  data collection 65
  treatment 121–2
authoring programs 131–2, **132**
automatic closed loop control 114
axial tomography 37

B-rep (boundary representation) systems
    118–19
backward-chaining systems 90, *91*
barcodes, optically scanned 4
BASIC 9, 82–3, 97
Baud rate 6–7, **7**
Bayes' theorem 83–7
  practical aspects 86–7
benchmark analysis 34
Bibliographic Retrieval Services (BRS)
    137–9
billing systems 17–18, 27–8

bitmap systems 87
blindness 116
bootstrapping 95
bottom-up systems 90
brain-injury, cognitive rehabilitation of
    117
British Journal of Healthcare Computing 26
BRS 137–9
BRS Colleague system 139
bulletin boards 140

C 9
Cancer Data Management System (CDMS)
    109
canonical phrase identification 69
cardiac pacemakers 120
CARE system 109, 135
carrier sense multiple access/collision
    detection (CSMA/CD) 8
cascade method 136
case-based systems 95
case mix index (CMI) 28
case mix management systems (CMM) 30
CASNET/GLAUCOMA 91
CBX 130
CD-ROM 132–3
CDC Wonder 140
charge-coupled device (CCD) camera 45–6
Chest Pain Study, multi-centre 104–5
clinical research information systems 75–6,
    77
Clinicom system 73
Clipper 10
COBOL 9
cochlea, artificial 116
cognitive prosthesis 107
collision detection 8
colour images 48
Common Basic Specification (CBS) 76
communications between computers 6–7
CompuServe 139
computed axial tomography (CAT-scans)
    50
computed radiography 50
computer-assisted design (CAD) 52

computer-assisted learning (CAL) 124–8,
  125
 acceptability of 128–9
 authoring programs 131–2, **132**
 benefits of 128
 bulletin boards 140
 distance learning 133
 drill-and-practice programs 124–6
 educational games 127–8
 educational philosophy 133–4
 efficacy of 129
 equipment required for 132–3
 factors restraining implementation of 129
 Hypertext 131
 medical dictionaries 136
 medical students and 135
 on-line medical information services
   136–40, **138–9**
 patient education and 134–5
 physicians and 135
 present and future role 134
 problem-solving programs 126
 programs for conducting tests 130
 reference retrieval 141
 simulation programs 127, **127**
 training staff in computer use 135–6
 tutorial programs 126
 video presentation 132, 133
 word processing and graphics 130–1, 133
computer-assisted manufacturing (CAM)
  52
computer-assisted medical decision making
  (CMD) 82–94, *84*
 defining the knowledge base 94–7
 design of 97–8
 domain-independent 97
 examples 102–5, **102**
 legal aspects 105–7
 performance assessment 98–102
  acceptability 102
  accuracy 99–100, **99**
  authority 101
  cost 101
  speed 101
  transferability 101
  usefulness 100–1
 presenting the findings 98
Computer Assisted Software Engineering
  (CASE) 34–5
computer-assisted soliloquy 120
computer based medical record (CBMR)
  54–77
 clinicians' reactions to 72
 data collection by 54–66
 examples 66–8, **67**
 patient reactions to 71–2
 staff involved in data input 68–9
 subjects suitable for 68–9
computer-based test interpretation (CBTI)
  77

computer models 76, 142–3
conferencing 140
confidentiality 65
congenital hypothyroidism (CHT)
  screening 111
Connection Machine 93
consequent-driven systems 90
constructive solid geometry (CSG) 118–19
COSTAR 66
costs
 of CMD system 101
 of computer-assisted learning 129
 of data collection system 66
 of database 140
 of installation 33
 projected, in UK 36
critical care 114
critical path analysis 31
critiquing 109
CSMA/CD 8
cue acquisition 91
cue interpretation 91
cueing 109

data access 74–5, **75**
data collection, computerised clinical 55–77
 advantages 62–5
 clinical research information systems 75–6
 collection by computer 55–60, *55*
  question design 56
  structured response 57, *57*, *58*
  types of question 55–6, **55**
  types of response 56–7
  validation by secondary questions 60
  validation of response 58–60
 data access 74–5
 data protection 73–4
 disadvantages 65–6
 initial design and organisation 61–2
 portable equipment 73
 prospective data 54, 61, 75
 questionnaire content 60–1
 retrospective data 54, 61, 75
 specialised data collection systems 77
 standardised questions 62, *63*
Data General 2
data models 76, 142–3
data-over-voice transmission 7
data protection 73–5
Data Protection Act (UK) 75
data reduction from medical equipment
  41–3, **42**
data transmission, clinical, standardisation
  of 146, **147**
database, choice of 140
database comparisons 87–8, *88*
database-management system (DBMS) 10
Dataease 10
daysheet 19
dBase IV 10

de Dombal system for abdominal pain 101, 103–4
deafness 116
DEC 2
decision analysis 111–13, *112*
decision threshold 112
decision tree 111, *112*
declarative knowledge 95
Delphic system 96
DERM/INFONET 140
desk top publishing (DTP) 131
diabetic management *46*, 120
diagnosis *see* medical diagnosis
diagnosis-related groups (DRGs) 28–9
Diagnostic Support System 96–7
DIALOG 137
digital filtration 38
digital imaging processing 46–8
digital signal 38
  automated analysis 38–41
DIOGENE 26
distance learning 133
DNA typing profiles 142
doctor-patient relationship, loss of 65
Doppler flow studies, use of colour in 48
DOS 4
dot-matrix printer 5–6
double-entry bookkeeping 19
Dr Spell 12
drill-and-practice programs 124–6
DXplain 104

educational games 127–8
educational philosophy 133–4
electrocardiography (ECG) 40, 41, 42–3
electronic mail 140
ELIZA program 120
EMYCIN 94
error traps 58–60
Ethernet network 8
Excerpta Medica 136, 137
exercise testing 43
expert systems 78
  application to clinical process 79, *80*
  in medical administration 32
expert systems shells 97

fast Fourier transform 40
floppy disk 132
Food, Drug and Cosmetic Act (FDCA) (USA) 106
foot operated switches 117
FORTRAN 9, 82
forward-chaining systems 90, *91*
Fourier analysis 39
Fourier transform (FT) 39–40, *40*
fourth generation languages 9
Foxpro 10
free-text processing 69
Freedom of Information Acts (USA) 75

frequency domain analysis 39–40
fuzzy set theory 87

general error traps 58, **59**
general ledger 19
Glasgow Coma Scale 100
grapevine transmission 7
graphical user interface (GUI) 4
graphics 131, 133
Griffiths Report 30
GUIDE 131

haematology 43
handicap 115–18
hardware 1–8
  breakdown 65–6
  communications between computers 6–7
  costs 33
  input devices 4–5
  large computer systems 3
  medium-size systems 2–3
  networking 7–8
  operating systems 4
  printers 5–6
  small computer systems 1–2
  smart cards 6
Harvard Graphics 131
health hazards
  of computer production 13
  of computer use 13, **14**
Health-Tex 135
high definition television (HDTV) 52
holography 118
Hospital Information Systems (HIS) 26, 27
Hounsfield numbers 50
Human Genome Project **144**
Hypercard 131
Hypermedia 131
Hypertext 131
hypothesis calculation 91
hypothesis generation 91

IBM 3
IBM-PC 1, 2
ICD system 144–6
ICD-9 29
ICD-9–CM 29
ICEM solid modeller 118
ICL 3
icons 5
Iliad 126
Image Management and Communication (IMAC) 51
image workstations 52–3
imaging 45–53, **47**
  automatic interpretation of images 53
  computed axial tomography (CAT-scans) 50
  computed radiography 50
  digital imaging processing 46–8

imaging (cont.)
  distribution of computerised images 51–2
  image densities 47–8, **48**
  image workstations 52–3
  improving image quality 48–50
    compression 49–50, 52
    enhancement 49, *49*
    noise reduction 49
    restoration 49
    subtraction 49, 53
  microscope images 53
  picture archiving and communication
    systems (PACS) 51
  presentation 48
  three-dimensional imaging 52
immunoassay 44
Index Medicus 137
Index of Health Education Micro-computer
    Programs 135
inductive systems 90
inference engine 85, 88
input devices 4–5
  ergonomic aspects 69
institutional database services 139
integrated circuit (IC) cards 6
Integrated Services Digital Network
    (ISDN) 7
INTERNET 133
INTERNIST (Caduceus) 103
Internist 97
INTERNIST-1 103
INTERNIST-1/QMR 126
IPA 7

JANET 133
joysticks 117

karyotyping 53
keyboards
  QWERTY 4, 69
  scanning 117
  specialised 5
knowledge base authors 82
knowledge engineers 82
Knowledge Index 137
Korner Report 29–30, 32

laboratory diagnosis 45, **45**
large computer systems 3
laser printers 5–6
Laservision 132
lightpens 4, 117
linear discriminant functions 87
LISP 97
liver biopsy 119
Logo 134

MACGEN 132
machine code 8
mainframe computers 3

management information systems 24
manufacturers, choice of 2
MD Computing 26
MEDELEXS 32
medical administration 16–36
  applications of computers 16–26, **17**
    financial management of health-care 17
      accounts 18–19
      billing systems 17–18, 27–8
      hospital finance department 20, **20**
      payroll 18, 32
      practice accounts 19–20
    general practice management 26
    Hospital Information Systems (HIS) 26,
      27
    patient appointment systems 24
    patient registers and indexes 20–1, **22**
    personnel selection 25–6
    pharmacy 22–4
      stock-control 22–3
    scheduling of facilities 25
    staff timetables 24–5
    stores and supplies 21–2
  expert systems 32
  installing a computer system 32–6, **34**
  management decisions in health care
      26–30
    clinical data collection 30
    resource management 26–7
      diagnosis-related groups (DRGs) 28–9
      private-sector management (USA) 27–8
      public-sector management (UK) 29–30
  management forecasting 30–2
medical diagnosis, computer-assisted
      78–107
  absolute vs operational diagnosis 81
  analytical vs synthetic
      (hypothetico-deductive) reasoning in
      81–2
  artificial intelligence (AI) 78–9, 94, **94**
  defining the knowledge base 94–7
  definition of diagnosis 79–80
  domain-independent CMD systems 97
  examples of CMD systems 102–5, **102**
  expert systems 78
  knowledge base as a Diagnostic Support
      System 96–7
  legal aspects of CMD systems 105–7
  methods 82–94, **83**
    algorithmic methods 82–3, *84, 89*
    cognitive models 91–3, *92*
    neural networks 93
    production rule systems 88–91, *89, 90*
    statistical pattern classification 83–8
  performance assessment of CMD
      systems 98–102
  self-diagnosis and self-treatment 105
  sharing knowledge bases 97
medical dictionaries 136
medical education 123–41

medical experts 82
Medical Information Bus 41
medical laboratory 44–5
medical management loop 109, *110*
Medical Special Interest Group (MedSIG) 139
medical terminology, standardisation of 143–6, **145**
Medical Writer 12
Medicare 28
Mediclip 131
medium-size systems 2–3
MEDLARS (MEDLINE) 136–7
MEDLINE 121, 136–7, 140
MedSIG 139
mental handicap 118
menus 5
MeSH 146
message error traps 58
Michelangelo virus 12
Microsoft Windows 4
MINET 139
minicomputers 2
Minnesota Multiphasic Personality Inventory (MMPI) 77
molecular biology, applications in 142
monitoring 109
Monte Carlo simulation techniques 142
mouse 5, 117
mouth sticks 117
MS-DOS 4
multiplexing 8
MYCIN 90–1, 94, 97

NASA 101
negative polarity 71
networking 7–8
neurocomputers 93
neurosurgery 119
nuclear medicine, use of colour in 48
nursing 121

Occam's razor 92, 97
Octree technique 118
off-line analysis 41
on-line analysis 41
on-line medical information services 136–40, **138–9**
ONCOCIN 91
Open Systems Interconnect (OSI) standards 7, 8
operating systems 4
operational requirement (OR) 35
optical cards 6
optical character reader (OCR) 130
optical mark readers 5
optically scanned barcodes 4
orthopaedics 119
Orthoplan 119
output devices, ergonomic aspects 69

pacemakers, cardiac 120
Paper Chase 139
Paradox 10
parallel processing 50
paralysed muscles, electrical stimulation of 117
paraplegia 117
Pascal 9, 82, 97
pathology laboratory 43–5
Patient Data Management System (PDMS) 114
Patient Data Query (PDG) system 139–40
patient registers and indexes 20–1, **22**
pattern matching 87
pattern recognition 93
payroll 18, 32
PCs 1–2
personnel selection 25–6
pharmacy 22–4
  stock-control 22–3
phenylketonuria (PKU) testing 111
picture archiving and communication systems (PACS) 51
pixel clutter 47
port-data output 41
pregnancy, use of VDU during 13
prescribing 114–15, *115*
printers 5–6
private-sector system of health care 27–8
problem knowledge coupler 92
procedural knowledge 95
program evaluation and review technique (PERT) 31
project management programs 31
PROLOG 97
prostheses, computer-driven 117
Psion 73
psychotherapy 120
public-sector system of health care 27, 29–30
PUFF 91, 97

QRS complex 40, 42
quadriplegia 117
Quattro 30
questionnaires 60–1
  self-administered 69
QUICK 96
QUICK MEDICAL REFERENCE (QMR) 87, 103
QWERTY keyboards 4, 69

radioimmunoassay 44
radiotherapy 113–14
reconstructive surgery 118–19
reference retrieval 141
regional mainframe 3
repetitve strain injury (RSI) 13
resource management 29
RS-232 serial port 41, 136

RxWRITER 114

scanning keyboard 117
screens
  design 70–1, *71*
  touch-sensitive 4, 117
screening programmes 111
Sears-Roebuck cluster 13
semen analysis 53
signal analysis 37–41
signal averaging 39
simulation programs 127, **127**
Sked-it 25
slow scan television (SSTV) 51
small computer systems 1–2
smart cards 6
SNA 7
SNOMED 144, 146
SNOP 144
software 8–12
  breakdown 65–6
  costs 33
  database packages 10
  errors, legal aspects 105–6
  fourth generation languages 9
  regulation of 106–7
  technical aspects of clinical database
    systems 10–11
  third generation languages 9
  turnkey systems 11–12
  wordprocessing 12
sound graphs 116
Soundex system 21
Source, The 139
specific error traps 58–60, **59**
speech recognition devices 72–3
speechlessness 116
sphygmomanometry 37
spreadsheets 30–1, **31**
statistical software packages 76, **77**
Stedman's Medical Dictionary 12
stereotactic procedures 119
structural query language (SQL) 11
study paradox 100
systems analysis 33

tactual vocoder 116
Tadoma method, synthetic 116
teleconferencing 133
telepresence surgery 119
Telxon systems 73
template analysis 41, *41*
terminals, siting of 69–70
Therac-25 incident 114
third generation languages 9
three-dimensional imaging 52
time domain analysis 38–9
time-flow analysis 24

time-sharing 8
time slice 8
TIME system 127
timetables 24–5
token-passing 8
top down systems 90
touch-sensitive screens 4, 117
training 35–6, 135–6
transducers 37, **38**
transparent error traps 58
treatment, computers and 108–22
  audit 121–2
  computers as medical prompts 108–9,
    110
  critiquing 109
  decision analysis 111–13, *112*
  nursing 121
  on-line database use 121
  specific areas 113–20, **113**
    anaesthesia 114
    cardiac pacemakers 120
    critical care 114
    diabetic management 120
    handicap 115–18
    orthopaedics 119
    prescribing 114–15
    psychotherapy 120
    radiotherapy 113–14
    reconstructive surgery 118–19
    stereotactic procedures 119
  in surveillance of medical action 109–11
  in surveillance of screening programmes
    111
turnkey systems 34
turns analysis 38
tutorial programs 126

Unified Medical Language (UML) 146
UNIX 4

varifocal mirror 118
VDU, hazards of use 13
vector processors 50
Veterans Administration 32
videodisc 132–3
virtual reality 119
viruses, computer 12
vision, artificial 116
voice volume and pitch detectors 117
voxels 118

Word 12
word processing 130
Wordperfect 12

XWindows 4

zero crossing 38